Bone Flaps in Reconstructive Surgery

Jayant P. Agarwal • David W. Mathes
Editors

Bone Flaps in Reconstructive Surgery

Anatomy and Technique

Springer

Editors
Jayant P. Agarwal
Division of Plastic Surgery
University of Utah School of Medicine
Salt Lake City, UT, USA

David W. Mathes
Division of Plastic and Reconstructive Surgery, Department of Surgery
University of Colorado Anschutz Medical Center
Aurora, CO, USA

ISBN 978-3-032-12539-2 ISBN 978-3-032-12540-8 (eBook)
https://doi.org/10.1007/978-3-032-12540-8

This Springer imprint is published by the registered company Springer Nature Switzerland AG
The registered company address is: Gewerbestrasse 11, 6330 Cham, Switzerland

Introduction

There are few textbooks in plastic surgery that focus on bony reconstruction, particularly the various options for vascularized bone flaps. Complex reconstructive procedures often require the re-establishment of multiple different tissue types. This includes bony reconstruction. Depending on the defect, bony reconstruction can require the use of vascularized bone flaps, particularly in larger defects or in suboptimal wound beds where bone grafts or substitutes will not take.

As plastic surgeons, we are involved in the reconstruction of all tissue types and are constantly identifying novel donor sites and flap options. We are taught that replacing like with like whenever possible is the optimal solution for any defect. This is especially true when rebuilding skeletal defects and re-creating the necessary hard tissue support. After trauma or tumor extirpation, reconstruction of the bony skeleton is fundamental to reestablishing a more normal form and function.

Bone defects that are of a critical size or that are associated with devascularized or radiated, or otherwise compromised, wound beds often need vascularized bone replacement for successful reconstruction.

As reconstructive surgeons, we often have preferred donor sites for soft tissue or bony reconstruction. As an example, our "go to" flap for bony reconstruction is the fibula when a vascularized segment of bone is required. This is mainly due to familiarity with the donor site and comfort with the dissection of the flap. The fibula offers versatility with regard to the amount of bone that can be harvested and vessel length, and it can be designed to include soft tissue for complex reconstructions.

It is often used for reconstruction of segmental defects or long bone stabilization as is seen in this example of a child with non-union after failed claviculo pro humeri reconstruction after osteosarcoma resection (Fig. 1) [1]. Here the fibula was used as an onlay to re-establish bony continuity and remodel with the residual humerus to provide a return of function.

Given its juxtaposition with the peroneal vessels and the robust vascular redundancy in the lower extremity, the fibula can also be used to reconstruct local defects as a pedicled flap. It has been pedicled locally to provide stability to or reconstruction of the nearby tibia, and it can also be used to reconstruct ankle defects when pedicled in a retrograde fashion via communicating branches between the posterior

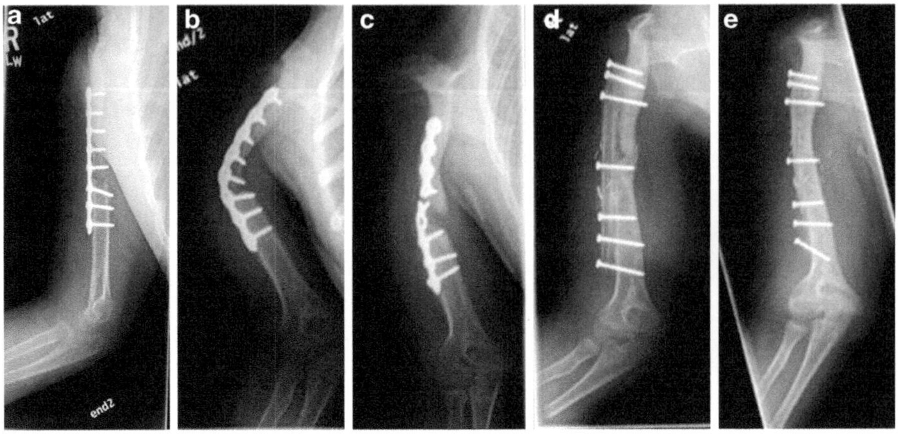

Fig. 1 Child with failed claviculo pro humeri after osteosarcoma resection. The free fibula flap was used as an onlay to re-establish bony continuity and ultimately remodeled with the humerus. (Reprinted [1])

tibial vessels and distal peroneal vessels (Fig. 2a and b) [2]. This case highlights the fibula's versatility in reconstructing the ankle syndesmosis in a young girl who had an osteosarcoma resected from the distal fibula.

Just as we have multiple options available for soft tissue reconstruction, it is beneficial for plastic surgeons to have a variety of vascularized bone options when tackling complex reconstructive cases. While the fibula flap can allow for bony reconstruction in a variety of scenarios including long bone, head and neck, or multi-segment reconstructions, there are several other options for vascularized bone that lend themselves to alternative or even more refined approaches to bony reconstruction. This is not to say that the fibula does not have its place as a leader in bony reconstruction.

In this textbook, we attempt to provide the plastic surgeon a variety of options for vascularized bone flaps. The hope is that plastic surgeons can utilize these alternative flaps as they are considering optimizing reconstructive outcomes for their patients. We have asked the world's leading experts on bone flaps and bony reconstruction to contribute chapters to this book. Each chapter offers anatomic description, surgical technique, and case examples for plastic surgeons to review and to ultimately use these flaps in their clinical cases.

This textbook highlights complex reconstructive scenarios where a variety of vascularized bone flaps are required. These range from complex head and neck reconstruction to extremity trauma or tumor extirpation to novel concepts in spinal reconstruction. The authors of these chapters have decades of experience refining their technique and innovating new procedures to optimize bone flap viability while minimizing donor site defects. As editors we have identified seasoned expert plastic surgeons as authors for each chapter. Additionally, you will note that each chapter is also authored by surgeons with new and different perspectives on the use of vascularized bone flaps.

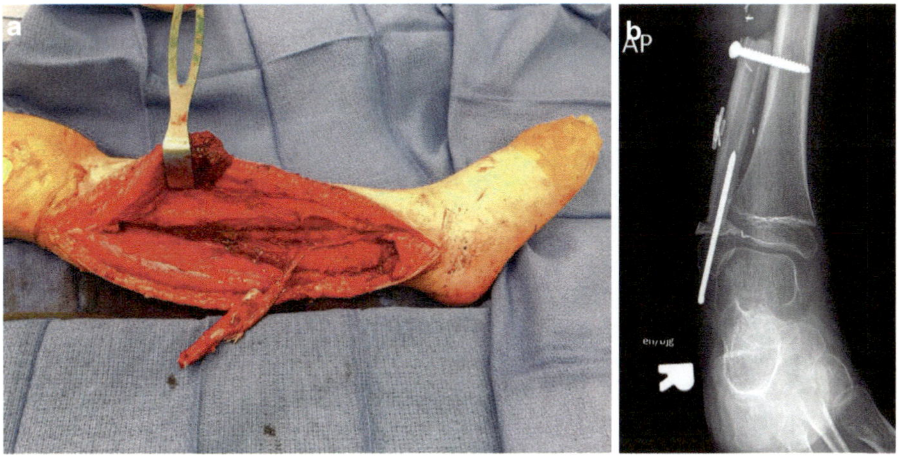

Fig. 2 (**a**, **b**) A child with distal fibula osteosarcoma resected. The proximal fibula is pedicled distally to reconstruct the ankle syndesmosis. (Reprinted [2])

Our hope is that plastic surgeons will learn alternative options for vascularized bone flaps and move outside of their comfort zone when tackling complex reconstructive challenges.

Division of Plastic Surgery
University of Utah School of Medicine
Salt Lake City, UT, USA
Jay Agarwal

Division of Plastic Surgery
University of Colorado School of Medicine
Aurora, CO, USA
David Mathes

References

1. Pires G, Moss WD, Luo J, Zhang R, Jones KB, Kwok AC, Agarwal JP. Free vascularized fibula salvage of failed CPH in pediatric sarcoma patients. Sarcoma. 2022 May 9.
2. Kwok AC, Tatro E, Jones KB, Agarwal JP. Pedicled retrograde fibula flap for ankle reconstruction after oncologic resection of the distal fibula. Plast Reconstr Surg Glob Open. 2017;5(2):e1232.

Contents

Contributors

Maureen Beederman Section of Plastic and Reconstructive Surgery, The University of Chicago Medicine & Biological Sciences, Chicago, IL, USA

Sarah M. Drejet Department of Otolaryngology – Head and Neck Surgery, University of Utah School of Medicine, Salt Lake City, UT, USA

Lawrence J. Gottlieb Section of Plastic and Reconstructive Surgery, The University of Chicago Medicine & Biological Sciences, Chicago, IL, USA

Matthew M. Hanasono Department of Plastic Surgery, The University of Texas MD Anderson Cancer Center, Houston, TX, USA

James Higgins Curtis National Hand Center, Medstar Union Memorial Hospital, Baltimore, MD, USA

Laura S. Humphries Division of Plastic and Reconstructive Surgery, University of Mississippi Medical Center, Jackson, MS, USA

Jason P. Hunt Department of Otolaryngology – Head and Neck Surgery, University of Utah School of Medicine, Salt Lake City, UT, USA

Z-Hye Lee Department of Plastic Surgery, The University of Texas MD Anderson Cancer Center, Houston, TX, USA

Jennifer Ling Department of Plastic and Reconstructive Surgery, Chang Gung Memorial Hospital, Taoyuan, Taiwan

Steven J. Lo Canniesburn Plastic Surgery Unit, Glasgow Royal Infirmary, Glasgow, UK
School of Medicine, Dentistry & Nursing, University of Glasgow, Glasgow, UK

Casey Martinez Alix School of Medicine, Mayo Clinic, Phoenix, AZ, USA

Evan Matros Memorial Sloan Kettering Cancer Center, New York, NY, USA

Ben C. McIntyre Division of Plastic and Reconstructive Surgery, University of Mississippi Medical Center, Jackson, MS, USA

Steven L. Moran Division of Plastic Surgery, Mayo Clinic, Rochester, MN, USA

Mohamed Morsy Department of Orthopaedic Surgery, The University of Alabama at Birmingham, Birmingham, AL, USA
Department of Orthopaedic Surgery, Assiut University Faculty of Medicine, Assiut University, Assiut, Egypt

Ledibabari Mildred Ngaage Department of Plastic and Reconstructive Surgery, Johns Hopkins School of Medicine, Baltimore, MD, USA

Jenny Lee Nguyen Texas Children's Hospital and Baylor College of Medicine, Houston, TX, USA

Danielle Olla Moffitt Cancer Center, Tampa, FL, USA

William C. Pederson Josephine Abercrombie Endowed Professor of Plastic Surgery, Baylor College of Medicine and Texas Children's Hospital, Houston, TX, USA
Surgery, Orthopedic Surgery, Neurosurgery, and Pediatrics, Baylor College of Medicine, Houston, TX, USA

Edward Reece Division of Plastic Surgery, Mayo Clinic, Phoenix, AZ, USA

Rou Wan Division of Plastic Surgery, Mayo Clinic, Rochester, MN, USA

Fu Chan Wei Department of Plastic and Reconstructive Surgery, Chang Gung Memorial Hospital, Taoyuan, Taiwan
Chang Gung University, Medical College, Taoyuan, Taiwan

Sebastian Winocour Department of Plastic Surgery, Baylor College of Medicine, Houston, TX, USA

Chapter 1
Fibula Free Flap

Ben C. McIntyre and Laura S. Humphries

Introduction and History

The fibula free flap is truly a workhorse flap for bone and combined bone and soft tissue reconstructions of the head and neck, limbs, and spine. Advantages include a reliable blood supply with readily available linear bone stock that can be contoured into a variety of configurations. Positioning also often lends itself well to a two-team approach and the donor site has acceptable morbidity for most patients. For extremity applications the diameter closely approximates that of the radius, ulna, and clavicle. It can also be "double-barreled" or inserted into large allografts for larger load-bearing bones such as the tibia and femur.

Many notable surgeons come to mind when discussing the history of the fibula free flap. *Taylor* et al. were the first to describe the fibula free flap and its use in the management of compound tibial fractures in 1975 [1]. In this early paper, the flap was used as a free osseous flap to reconstruct bone gaps in the mid/distal tibia in two patients. These straight bone struts were "doweled" into the proximal and distal tibia. Prior to these transfers, Taylor performed multiple angiographic and cadaveric studies confirming the dominant pedicle of the peroneal artery. He described an artery of 1.8 mm in diameter and two venae comitantes, 2–4 mm in diameter. Shortly thereafter, in 1989, *Hidalgo* published his results of 12 patients undergoing segmental mandibulectomy and reconstruction with a fibula flap [2]. Noted advancements included osteotomies to create a naturally shaped mandible and mini-plate fixation. A cutaneous skin paddle was carried with the flap based on a septocutaneous perforator in 5 patients. Of these, only 1 skin paddle had 100% take which the author cited as a major drawback. By 1999, *Cordeiro* et al. *(of which Hidalgo was a co-author)* had published a series of 135 fibula flaps for mandibular reconstruction

B. C. McIntyre (✉) · L. S. Humphries
Division of Plastic and Reconstructive Surgery, University of Mississippi Medical Center, Jackson, MS, USA

J. P. Agarwal, D. W. Mathes (eds.), *Bone Flaps in Reconstructive Surgery*,
https://doi.org/10.1007/978-3-032-12540-8_1

with 100% success and 90% skin paddle survival [3]. Clearly, the reliability of the skin paddle had been established. Throughout the 1990s many advancements had been made including osseointegration, skin paddle design, and operative decision-making [4–7]. Fu Chan Wei cannot be omitted in this discussion as he and his group in Taiwan have made many contributions to the understanding of the fibula blood supply and anatomy, as well as innovations such as the double-barrel flap and jaw in a day surgery [8–15].

Indications

The decision to use a vascularized bone graft (VBG) in reconstructive surgery can seem straightforward but it is important to review surgical indications as the option for nonvascularized bone grafts (NVBGs) may be warranted in some patients with smaller segmental defects. Vascularized osteocutaneous flaps should be considered in any defect requiring both bone and soft tissue reconstruction, radiated wounds, or in salvage cases in which NVBG failed [16]. Often the patient's age and comorbidities may guide the surgeon to consider NVBG or even a pedicled flap reconstruction (e.g., pectoralis major musculocutaneous flap in the infirm head and neck patient). A word of caution in the latter situation is that often if an elderly patient can tolerate a pectoralis major flap, then they likely can tolerate a fibula free flap in the hands of a skilled microsurgeon.

Bone union rates are generally much higher in VBG versus NVBG. In the previously cited study by Foster et al. they reported a VBG union rate of 96% versus NVBG of 69% in those patients undergoing mandibular reconstruction following segmental resection [16]. Pogrel et al. reported similar findings in the head and neck citing a 95% union rate in VBG patients versus a 76% success rate in NVBG [17]. In the lower extremity Yazar et al. reported the experience from Chang Gung Hospital having a long bone union rate of 88.9% with VBG with an average union time of 6.9 months. Capanna et al. reported their long-term follow-up of patients undergoing vascularized fibula with massive bone allograft for femur and tibia reconstructions and had a 93.5% union rate versus an 80% union rate with allograft alone [18].

For head and neck reconstruction the indications for VBG are:

- Composite defects with bone gaps ≥6 cm.
- Smaller defects (<6 cm) requiring a skin island for mucosal reconstruction.
- Radiated wound beds (preoperative or postoperative radiation).
- Salvage cases with failure of NVBG.
- Cases in which osseointegrated implants are planned.
- Blast injuries with a heavily traumatized wound bed.

Extremity indications for VBG are not as clearly defined as they are in the head and neck applications. Orthopedic surgeons are more familiar with large nonvascular bone allografts and bone transport with distraction osteogenesis than VBG and it is likely that this technique is underutilized in this patient population. Advantages to VBG over bone transport in the extremity include immediate plate fixation, wound closure, and avoidance of an external frame during a prolonged period of bone transport [18]. Long-term data supporting VBG can be garnered from the Taylor et al. 2016 report of extensive VBG [19]. In 384 cases he reported a 95% success rate with a time to union in the upper limb of 8–10 weeks and in the lower limb of 3–4 months. We feel that VBG in extremity reconstruction is likely underutilized and should be considered as part of the algorithm for patients with extremity skeletal defects.

Our recommendations for extremity VBG include:

- Composite defects with segmental bone loss >6 cm and soft tissue/skin loss.
- Radiated wound beds such as in the case of soft tissue or bone malignancies.
- Failed allograft or nonunions following standard orthopedic fixations, especially in patients with tenuous skin coverage.
- Cases of chronic osteomyelitis in which limb salvage is an option.
- Blast injuries with a damaged wound bed.

Situations in which VBG has been used in the pelvis, spine, hand, foot, and clavicle are less well defined as there have only been case reports or small series describing the use of the fibula flap in these locations. For these clinical situations, the authors recommend expanding the above indications individually to the given patient.

Surgical Anatomy

When raising a fibula free flap, the surgeon must have mastered the anatomy of the lower extremity including the anatomic compartments of the calf and their contents (Fig. 1.1). All three primary vessels (posterior tibial, anterior tibial, and peroneal arteries) to the lower limb will be identified during the dissection. Additionally, all four compartments of the lower limb will be identified and opened during exposure. The peroneal nerve and its branches will need to be identified and protected during the dissection.

The fibula free flap is a Mathes and Nahai Type V flap with a dominant pedicle and several segmental vascular pedicles which arise from the anterior tibial and posterior tibial vessels [20–22]. For procedural purposes, the flap will be raised on the peroneal artery and its venae commitantes [1, 21–24]. The minor segmental perforators only become important if the proximal epiphysis is to be transferred [22]. The classic anatomical description of the popliteal artery branch pattern is that at the neck of the fibula the popliteal artery bifurcates into the anterior and posterior tibial arteries (the latter of which forms the tibioperoneal trunk) [22]. The peroneal artery branches off of the tibioperoneal trunk at a variable distance (usually 1–3 cm). A short tibioperoneal trunk will mean a longer vascular pedicle and vice versa. This branching pattern is present in 79% of patients [22]. An important anatomic variable

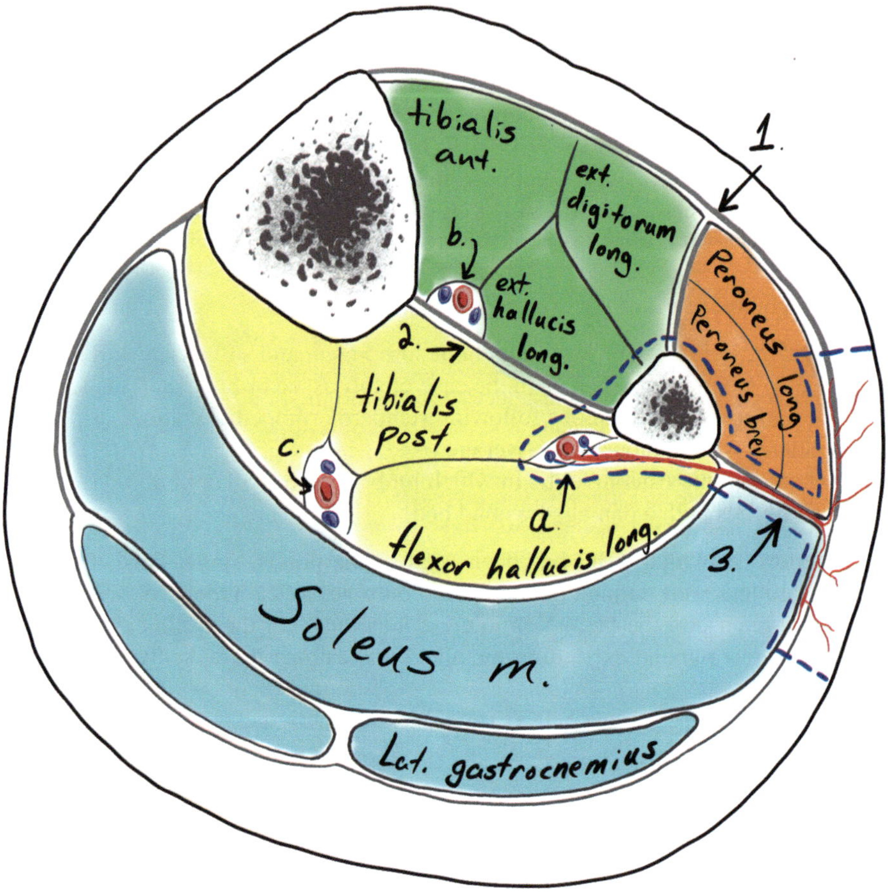

Fig. 1.1 Cross-sectional anatomy of the tibia and fibula. Compartments: orange—lateral compartment, green—anterior compartment, yellow—deep posterior compartment, light blue—superficial posterior compartment. Vasculature: (a) peroneal artery, (b) anterior tibial artery, (c) posterior tibial artery. Septae: (1) anterior intermuscular septum, (2) interosseous membrane, (3) posterior intermuscular septum. Dark blue dotted line—fibula flap dissection planes to include peroneal vascular pedicle

is the single dominant peroneal artery or peronea magna which is present in up to 2% of patients [22].

The flap generally will need to be harvested near the takeoff from the posterior tibial artery in order to maximize pedicle length. In anatomic studies, the mean length of the vascular pedicle is 11.15 cm and the mean arterial diameter is 2.83 mm [25]. Typically two veins of varying size can be found accompanying the artery with an average diameter of 3.51 mm [25]. Bone perfusion occurs through a nutrient artery and multiple periosteal branches emanating directly from the peroneal artery. Most nutrient arteries enter the fibula at the middle third with an average distance from the proximal fibula head to the foramina of 14.1 cm [26]. Ninety percent of patients will have a single nutrient artery with a foraminal opening of 1.2 mm (0.9–1.5 cm) [26].

The fibula bone in cross section is a triangular-shaped bone with a mean length of 33.1 cm [25]. This cross-sectional diameter nearly mirrors that of the radius, ulna, and clavicle [22]. Given that approximately 6–8 cm of bone on both the proximal and distal ends of the fibula will be preserved during flap harvest, approximately 17–21 cm of bone will be available for contouring and positioning. The lateral surface is generally the flattest part of the fibula and lends itself well to plating.

Several muscles of importance originate from the fibula. The peroneus longus and brevis muscles in the lateral compartment attach to the anterolateral surfaces of the fibula. The soleus muscle and flexor hallucis longus (FHL) originate from the posterolateral surface of the fibula. The FHL is particularly susceptible to injury as it will usually be completely dissected free of its originations. Injury to this muscle or failure to reattach it to the surrounding soft tissues during donor site closure can cause claw toe due to unopposed action of the extensor hallucis longus muscle [27].

The peroneal nerve along with the deep and superficial branches will be exposed during the course of the dissection. The common peroneal nerve arises from the sciatic nerve in the popliteal fossa and sweeps around the fibular head beneath the peroneus longus muscle. In this region it branches into the superficial peroneal nerve which enters the lateral compartment and innervates the peroneus longus and brevis muscles. The final ramifications of this nerve can be seen distally exiting the lateral compartment and providing sensory innervation to the distal lateral calf and the dorsum of the foot. The deep peroneal nerve enters the anterior compartment and innervates all anterior compartment muscles with its final ramification providing sensation to the first webspace of the foot. These nerves must be carefully protected during flap elevation. Injury to the superficial peroneal nerve will cause loss of foot eversion and dorsal foot anesthesia, while injury to the deep branch will cause loss of foot dorsiflexion and first webspace anesthesia.

Peroneal Artery Skin Territory and Designing an Osseofasciocutaneous Flap

The peroneal artery gives 4–5 perforators to the skin surface which are either septocutaneous from the posterior intermuscular septum or musculocutaneous [22]. Proximally, these perforators tend to be musculocutaneous as they course through the lateral gastrocnemius and soleus muscles. These perforators generally are distributed segmentally at intervals 2–6 cm from each other [23]. Anatomic studies by Wei et al. have demonstrated a skin perforator diameter of 0.8–1.7 mm as they exit the posterior intermuscular septum [23]. This group also reported a possible skin paddle length of 25 cm and a width of 14 cm when the flap is centered over the posterior fibular margin at the junction of the middle and distal thirds of the fibula [23]. Mathes and Nahai have reported a possible skin territory of 8 × 15 cm [21].

In an important clinical anatomic study by Yu and Hanasono, 80 patients were studied at that time of fibula flap harvest for cutaneous perforator location [28]. They found 1–3 perforators clustered over the third quarter of the fibula at a line 1–1.5 cm posterior to the long axis of the fibula. Forty-nine percent had a single perforator and 36% had two perforators. Ninety-six percent were septocutaneous perforators over this distal location. A more proximal perforator was reliably found in 70 patients on average 11.9 cm ± 1.9 cm from the fibular head. The distal perforator cluster is critical for skin paddle perfusion over the fibula. The more proximal perforator is most useful when a secondary skin paddle is required, such as in the event of when both intraoral and extraoral defects are made in head and neck procedures.

Skin perforator localization is done by the authors prior to prepping the leg in the operating room [29]. The proximal fibular head and lateral malleolus are marked on the skin and then the longitudinal axis of the fibula is transposed on the skin. At the junction of the middle and distal thirds of the fibula, about 1 cm posterior to the long axis line, handheld doppler exam is used to mark the skin perforators. The skin paddle can then be reliably oriented on this perforator. If a second skin paddle is desired, then proximal Dopplering is done based on the perforator mapping study done by Yu and Hanasono noted above [28]. It is important for the surgeon to know that the septocutaneous perforators always travel along the posterior surface of the fibula. This is critical when elevating the flap in that the dissection over the anterior surface of the fibula in the lateral and anterior compartments can be done quickly without worry that the septocutaneous skin perforator will be damaged during this step. The authors also typically elevate the skin paddle on the deep fascia of the leg in order to provide more reliable perfusion to the skin surface. If possible, the skin paddle can also be planned around areas that are devoid of hair, especially if an intraoral skin paddle is planned. If primary skin closure of the skin paddle defect is not possible, then it is advisable that the skin paddle not be oriented over the lateral malleolus as this is a common area of thin soft tissue. This is done to prevent an open wound and exposed bone at the lateral malleolus.

Choosing a Limb Donor Site and Pedicle Orientation

The versatility of the fibula flap cannot be overemphasized. Its long pedicle can usually reach both sides of the neck in contralateral reconstructions. The artery is of good caliber and can be anastomosed to a variety of recipient vessels including the facial, superficial temporal, and superior thyroid artery. The veins can also be large enough to match well with the external jugular vein and facial vein and can also be easily anastomosed end to side to the internal jugular vein.

When deciding upon the laterality of a fibula flap harvest, a detailed physical exam of the lower extremities is always a good starting point. Normal pedal pulses should always be palpable. If not, documentation of the handheld Doppler signals of the pedal pulses is also important. Signs of ischemic leg disease such as hair loss, smooth shiny skin, and cool toes should be evaluated and documented. The clinician should also look for signs of prior trauma, incisions, fractures, and evidence of venous stasis and lymphedema. The patient's gait and use of a cane or walker should also be noted. A small factor in the decision to use one leg over the other may also be that US drivers tend to use their right foot more frequently.

The CTA can give you valuable information on which leg you may choose to use. We obtain these on every patient given the chances for a normal vascular exam in the anomaly of peronea magna (single peroneal artery to the foot). Now that VSP is commonplace, high-resolution imaging of the fibula is important for anatomic planning, hence another reason to order this on every patient. The information garnered from the CT scan should detail the presence of one-, two-, or three-vessel runoff to the foot. The presence of intraluminal calcifications should also be noted especially in the areas of the proximal pedicle and areas of tight osteotomies. Pipestem vessels do not flex much around acute pedicle turns. There may also be a long tibioperoneal trunk on one side which would effectively shorten the pedicle. Varicosities and signs of incompetent dilated deep veins of the leg should be evaluated. Signs of prior trauma such as fractures and bullet fragments should also be looked for on the CTA.

Most reconstructions can be designed off either leg depending on the scenario. Plans can be made with the vascular pedicle trailing off the anterior aspect of the intended reconstruction (e.g., anterior body toward the symphysis) or with the vascular pedicle descending into the neck off the posterior aspect of the reconstruction (e.g., toward the angle). When performing ramus, condyle, and body reconstructions, it is best to have the pedicle extend off the anterior edge of the reconstruction to prevent an acute turn of the pedicle up near the condyle back into the upper neck. This will shorten and compromise the pedicle if this is done.

When planning a fibula flap it is important to be cognizant of several key points. The first is that the skin paddle when the flap is elevated will hang from the lower lateral aspect of the fibula flap. The second is that plating will be on the lateral side of the fibula. Based on this four-flap configurations could be possible. The first example would be vessels extending posterior from an ipsilateral fibula flap. The flap can be transferred up to the body with the plate on the lateral aspect of the flap and the skin paddle will rotate up and over the plate on what would be the buccal side of the flap. The second example would be vessels extending from the anterior (symphyseal) border of an ipsilateral flap. In this situation with an ipsilateral body reconstruction, the flap would turn 180° along its long axis bringing the skin paddle from the inferior to superior position in the mouth and the vascular leash anteriorly. The plate would still lie on the flat lateral surface of the fibula.

Keeping with the same recipient area of the body of the mandible, the contralateral fibula could be used. With the contralateral leg and the intended direction of the vascular pedicle posteriorly the flap will rotate 180° on its short axis which will bring the flat lateral surface of the fibula flap to the contralateral buccal side of the mandible and also will bring the skin paddle superiorly into the mouth. The fourth scenario would be if the vessels were to be anterior from a contralateral flap toward the symphysis. The flap would rotate 180° on its long axis and 180° on its short axis. The former effect would bring the vessels anterior and the skin paddle superior, the

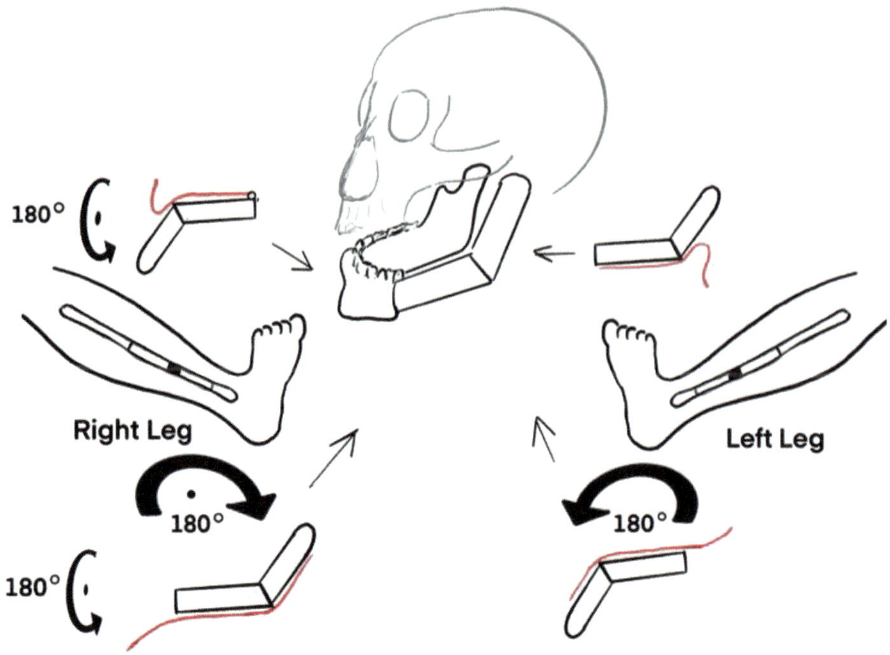

Fig. 1.2 Potential orientation and rotation schematics of multiple fibula flap configurations from opposite legs using vessels for anteriorly or posteriorly flap orientation configurations

latter effect would bring the smooth plating surface back lateral, and the skin paddle would now be hanging from the inferior aspect of the flap. This means the skin island would swing up and over the plate along the buccal side into the intraoral location as it did in the first scenario (Fig. 1.2).

The authors understand this can be confusing but models and preoperative planning can help avoid the intraoperative pitfall of not knowing how the skin island is going to be oriented. A larger skin paddle should be considered in the first series of patients for most surgeons as this will allow for more flexibility in skin paddle orientation should the skin paddle not rotate or inset as planned. The excess can always be trimmed away and the donor site grafted. A last pearl is that the skin paddle has difficulty rotating into the lingual side of the flap because the tight space of the surrounding tissues such as the remnant tongue and vascular pedicle can constrict the pedicle and lead to venous congestion.

Virtual Surgical Planning (VSP)

Virtual surgical planning has revolutionized head and neck reconstruction with the fibula flap. Through conventional high-resolution CT scans, patient-specific data can be uploaded into various software bundles allowing for precise estimation of the surgical defect and precise design of cutting guides and reconstruction plates. This has enabled the creation of complex geometrical fibula flap shapes in the case of orbitozygomaticomaxillary reconstructions, double-barreled flap configurations and jaw in a day surgery utilizing precise placement of osseointegrated dental implants (Fig. 1.3a, b). A variety of models and cutting guides can be generated and sterilized to aid the surgeon during the procedure which saves times and improves precision (Fig. 1.4a, b). Also from this data, precontoured reconstruction plates can be designed and milled according to the surgeon's specifications.

Fibula cutting guides come in two main types, nylon/acrylic and titanium. Both types are equally precise, but the nylon/acrylic models have a shorter turnaround time of 7–10 days, in urgent cases, than the titanium guides (currently around 14 days). Titanium guides have the advantage of a lower profile when positioned on the fibula which aids visualization of the bone and vascular pedicle during contouring by the surgical team. This is also an added benefit when teaching residents on surgical technique as both teacher and learner have improved visualization of critical structures. Both types of guides will have narrow slots in them which allow for the passing of oscillating or reciprocating saws to make precise osteotomies. There will be biplanar fixation holes which will be used to screw anchor the guide to the fibula during contouring. These temporary screws should be unicortical. The authors perform the fibula contouring after the fibula flap is fully elevated but still tethered by its pedicle to the lower limb, minimizing ischemia time. The authors also perform 80–90% osteotomy cuts with the cutting guide in place and then remove the guide as the osteotomies are completed. This is done so that the vascular pedicle can be seen clearly during the final portion of this critical step.

When designing a fibular cutting guide during VSP sessions, the authors typically place the distal osteotomy around 7 cm from the lateral malleolus. This allows

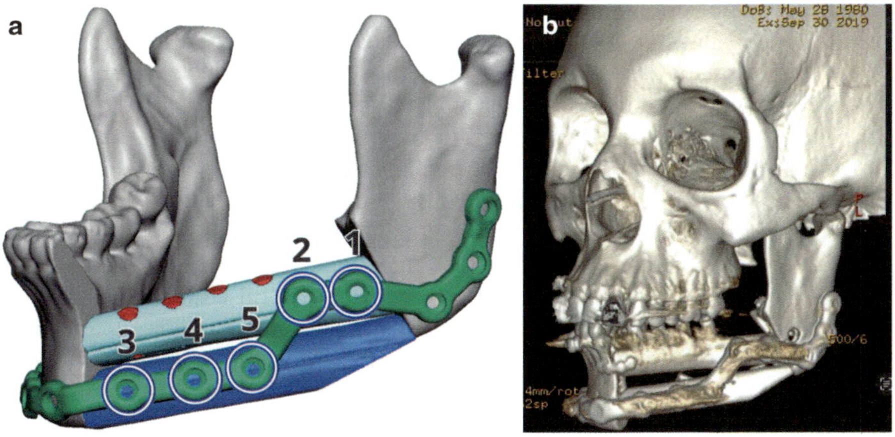

Fig. 1.3 (**a**, **b**) Example of a double barrel fibula flap segmental body reconstruction with osseointegrated implants. (**a**) VSP mockup, (**b**) Postop CT scan. Note miniplate used to secure the superior bone segment to the symphysis

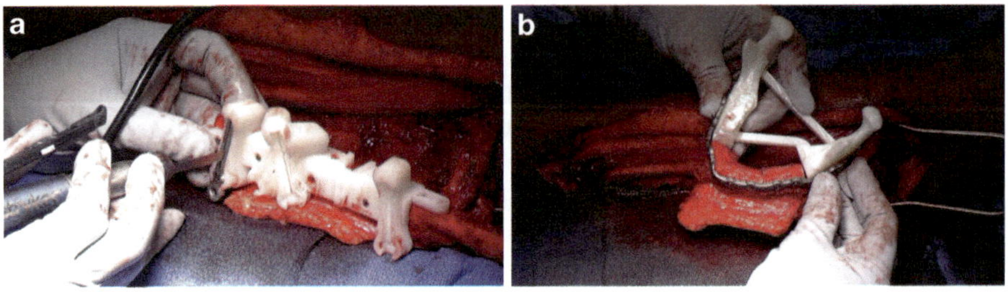

Fig. 1.4 (**a**) Intraoperative view of a fibula cutting guide in place on the lateral aspect of the fibula. (**b**) Plated three-segment fibula flap for mandible reconstruction using VSP

for maximization of pedicle length as the flap is elevated. The guide can always be shifted proximally for fit and skin paddle location. Drawbacks of these cutting guides are that the fibula skin paddle perforator location is generally not known when the planning session is done. This makes precise planning of the skin paddle arc of rotation more difficult. Another drawback is that the soft tissue bulk surrounding the fibula (the typical 1–3-mm cuff of muscle offset) can make fit of the guide loose or not as anatomic as was done during the computer-generated session. Small deviations from the original plan can lead to bone gaps and poor fit of the bone graft into the recipient site, so added care must be taken when affixing the guide to the fibula.

Common larger mandibular reconstructions can usually be done with three segments of bone. For instance, an angle to angle reconstruction can be done with two body segments on either side of a symphysis segment. A hemimandible from condyle to symphysis can be done with a ramus, body, and symphysis segment. For most surgical applications this will be the most bone that you need and the fibula on an average-sized person will have ample length of bone available.

When planning osteotomies, fibula bone segments should typically be no smaller than 1-2 cm to allow for good segmental periosteal blood supply reaching the bone. If a double-barreled flap is planned, a 1–2-cm wedge of bone should be removed from between the osteotomy segments to allow for a more gentle arc of rotation for the pedicle as it makes a 180° turn to run the opposite direction.

During the planning sessions, a design for the placement of osseointegrated implants can be done. The surgeons and design team will need to take into account the location of the plate fixation screws anchoring the fibula bone segments in place to avoid hardware contact and malalignment. Other adjustments that are typically made during VSP for implant placement are to raise the fibula flap bone segments to a more superior location nearing the remnant mandible superior cortex which brings the implants closer to the occlusal plane. It is important to note that an implant is not needed for each tooth that is removed as multiple implants drilled into the fibula will weaken it and can lead to iatrogenic fracture. Two to three implant posts for a unilateral dental restoration are plentiful to create stability and prevent "wobble" of a partial dental prosthesis that will be anchored to them.

Condylar shaping using VSP is also extremely precise. Patients can differentiate when their occlusion is off by as much as 1 mm so it very important to get these measurements as accurate as possible. The VSP technicians can often overlay a mirror image of the condyle over the reconstruction and use this to design a separate jig for contouring what will be the articular surface of the neocondyle. Our group has found it best to err on the side of making the reconstructed ramus segment slightly shorter by 2–3 mm in these instances in order to allow the contralateral dentition to make premature contact. As is often the case in these reconstructions, the contralateral teeth are the only teeth remaining for grinding/chewing of food so this is very important.

Virtual surgical planning has rapidly supplanted hand carving of fibula flaps in head and neck cases. Outcomes and cost benefits must be weighed carefully when considering the added expense of this technology. In a large meta-analysis by Pucci et al., VSP-designed fibula flaps demonstrated more accuracy in intercondylar distances (2.0 vs. 3.9 mm) and gonial angles (3.6° vs. 7.7°) when compared to traditional hand cutting techniques [30]. This same study also found a decrease in mean ischemia time to 73.8 min (VSP) versus 109.9 minutes (hand carved) and reduction in total operative mean time to 391.8 min (VSP) versus 457.6 min (hand carved). A similar meta-analysis by Tang et al. also demonstrated significantly decreased operative times (standardized mean difference −1.01; 95% CI −1.23 to 0.80; $p = 0.000$), ischemia times (standardized mean difference −1.55; 95% CI −1.87 to −1.23, $p = 0.002$), and improved orthognathic outcomes when compared to traditional hand-carved fibula flaps [31]. Added cost is also a consideration when VSP is utilized. Mazzola et al. from Sydney Head and Neck Unit reported a shorter median length of stay (10.0 vs. 13.0 days, $p = 0.009$), lower mean procedure time (507.38 vs. 561.75 min, $p = 0.042$), and lower mean total cost ($35,493 vs $37,345) when comparing VSP-designed to traditional reconstructions [32]. In a recent paper out of MD Anderson, Kurlander et al. have demonstrated that despite an average increased additional cost of $10,400 for the patient, improved outcomes of quality-adjusted life years in metrics such as speech quality, likelihood of returning to a regular diet, better occlusion, and decreased nonunions suggested that this technology vastly outweighed the upfront cost of the technology [33]. Given improvements in length of stay, quality of life, diminished operative, and ischemia times, the authors agree that VSP should be considered the standard of care with more complex reconstructions.

Surgical Technique

Positioning and Room Setup: The fibula flap is best raised and inset using a two-team approach when possible. In the preoperative area it is best to reconfirm the laterality, review the CT angiogram, and go over the operative plan with the patient. Once in the operating room, the patient is positioned supine with a slight bump under the hip if possible. A lateral approach to the fibula is preferred. For head and neck cases the table usually is turned 180° for ease of positioning the microscope and instrument tables. A sterile tourniquet will also be used.

Preoperative Markings: Markings are done prior to prepping of the critical landmarks which are the proximal and distal fibular heads (Fig. 1.5). The proximal fibular head is palpated just distal to the knee flexion crease and there is usually a soft groove beneath the skin that the fingers can roll over indicating the most proximal extent of the fibula. The distal fibular head/lateral malleolus is similarly marked. A longitudinal line is then drawn on the skin overlying the long shaft of the fibula. This line will connect the proximal and distal fibular heads. A ruler is used to measure the distance of the long axis of the fibula flap and the total length recorded. This distance should be divided by 3 and the fibula long axis divided into thirds. This is marked on the skin. At the juncture of the distal and middle thirds of the fibula is where the most distal skin perforator is most reliably identified. The perforator often will enter through the lateral crural septum which will be about 1 cm posterior to the palpable axis of the fibula. The perforator generally will be within 3 cm of this landmark. Additional perforators should be Dopplered proximally in the event that a larger skin paddle or multiple skin paddles are required. A template of the skin/mucosa defect should be oriented over this distal perforator.

Initial Flap Dissection: This has been published previously [29]. The flap is preferably elevated under an above knee tourniquet at 300 mmHg. The flap should be able to be elevated within 2 h. The leg is not exsanguinated in order to facilitate visualization of the perforators. The initial skin incision is made extending from just a few cm proximal to the lateral malleolus, then along the anterior border of the skin paddle, and then proximally up to the proximal fibular head. This incision is

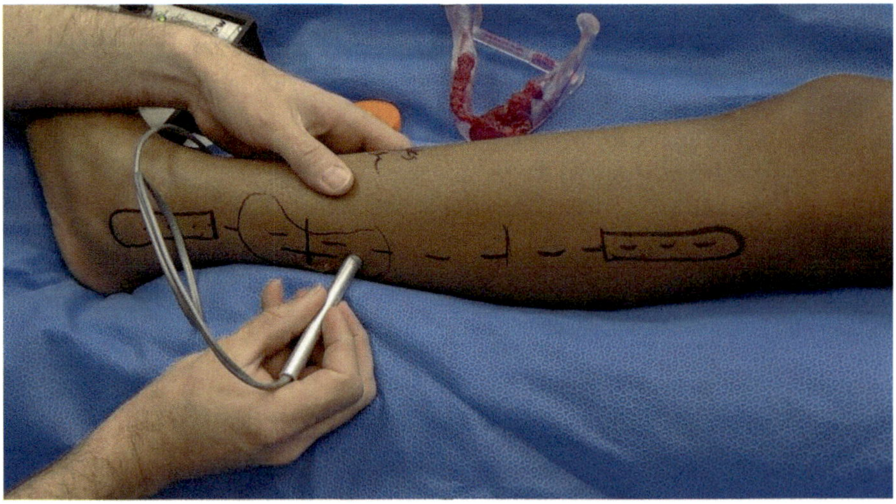

Fig. 1.5 Surgical markings for the fibula flap. The proximal fibular head and lateral malleolus are marked. A line is drawn along the long axis of the fibula and Doppler perforator markings are made along the juncture of the middle and distal thirds of the fibula

deepened to the deep muscle fascia and the fascia along the anterior edge of the skin paddle is incised and the dissection is carried posteriorly to the lateral intermuscular septum. The perforator to the skin paddle should be visualized within this septum. Once the skin perforators are identified, the skin paddles can be adjusted accordingly.

Deep Muscular Dissection: With the perforators identified and skin paddles designed, the fibula flap can be mobilized, compartment by compartment. The lateral compartment muscles (peroneus longus and brevis) will be encountered first. Using Bovie cautery, these muscles are taken off the fibula in a distal to proximal direction. It is important to leave a 1–2-mm muscle cuff on the fibula to give some soft tissue protection to the fibula in the event of an oral mucosal separation. As the muscles are reflected anteromedially, the bone will become more and more exposed. During this step the superficial peroneal nerve will be seen within a fat stripe of the peroneus muscles. This nerve is best mobilized with bipolar cautery.

The anterior intermuscular septum is then incised and the anterior compartment entered. It is important to keep close to the deep surface of the fibula to avoid injury to the anterior compartment neurovascular structures. The anterior tibial vessels and deep peroneal nerve should be readily visualized during this step. The nerve should be carefully protected as the anterior compartment muscle structures are taken off the fibula. Proximally, the surgeon will see the deep and superficial peroneal nerves join to become the common peroneal nerve. It is at the proximal fibular head that the common branch is most susceptible to iatrogenic injury. The authors prefer to mobilize the peroneal nerve almost to the proximal fibular head so that it can be reflected out of the way during the fibular osteotomies.

At this juncture the remainder of the dissection will be hampered until the proximal and distal fibular osteotomies are made (Fig. 1.6). To maintain ankle and knee

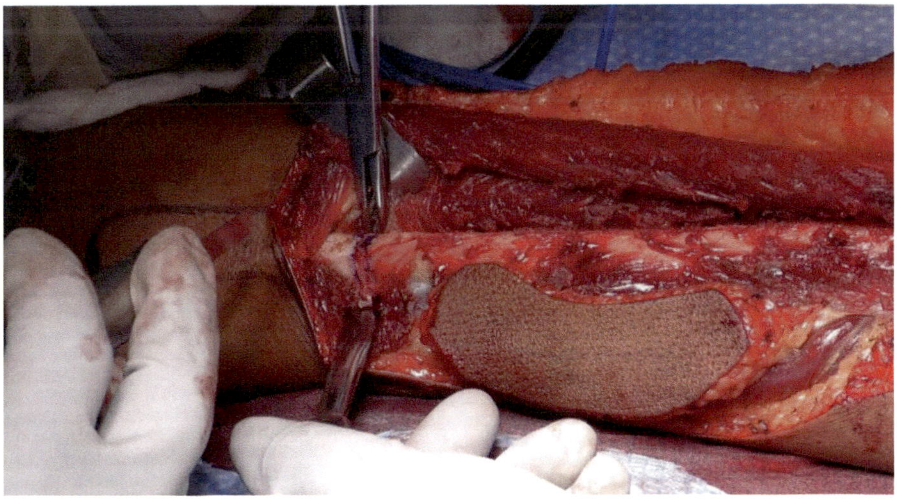

Fig. 1.6 Fibular osteotomies are made with an oscillating saw. Care is taken to protect the vascular pedicle which lies just deep to the bone

stability, it is important to keep 7–8 cm of bone on either end of the fibula. At the intended osteotomy sites, periosteal elevators are used to make a zone for these bone cuts. At the distal osteotomy site, a right angle, Hohmann, or Army Navy retractor is passed along the back of the fibula and used as a stop to protect the pedicle (the peroneal artery/vein). A 10-mm oscillating saw is used to make the first cut. A small wafer of bone is best removed at this site also to allow for more mobility of the fibula. The proximal fibular osteotomy is made in a similar fashion, but utmost care should be taken to protect the peroneal vascular pedicle proximally when making this proximal osteotomy.

With the proximal and distal osteotomies made, the fibula should start to become very mobile. Place bone clamps on the bone to aid in lateral retraction and then open the interosseous membrane. Distally, the peroneal vessels should be visible nearly immediately after opening this membrane (Fig. 1.7). The distal end of the pedicle is doubly clipped and ligated. The plane of dissection will now be in the deep compartment and will extend proximally. The critical mark at this juncture will be the flexor hallucis longus (FHL) muscle which has a houndstooth appearance from its bipennate anatomy. This muscle will be opened up and just deep to it will be the peroneal vascular pedicle. The posterior tibial vessels will be also visualized medial to the pedicle. Multiple interconnecting small muscular branches will be seen going between these vessels and will need to be clipped and ligated.

Final Steps of Flap Mobilization: As the flap is further dissected proximally, the remaining muscular attachments of the FHL will be taken down. If not already done, the skin paddles should be islanded and the superficial posterior compartment muscles (soleus and lateral gastrocnemius) will be taken off the fibula. Proximally, one can commonly find a perforator entering the lateral gastrocnemius or soleus

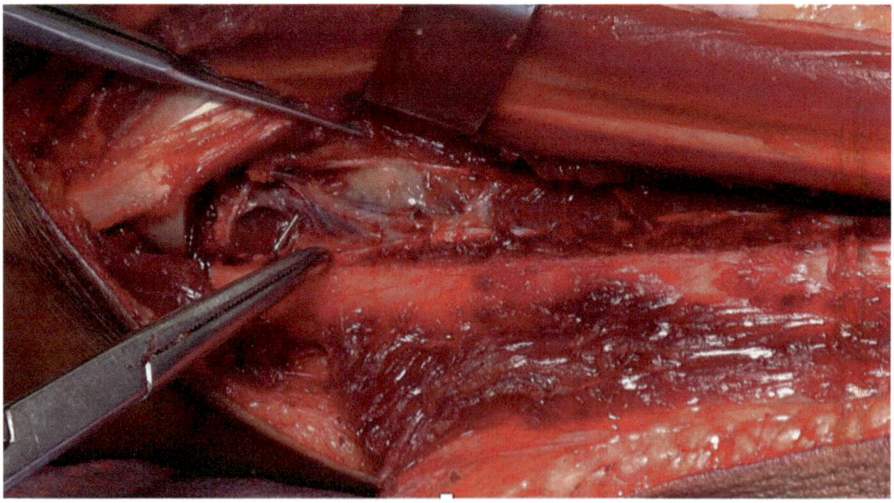

Fig. 1.7 The distal peroneal artery vascular pedicle is identified just deep to the fibula and the interosseous membrane. It is doubly clipped and divided distally as the flap is mobilized

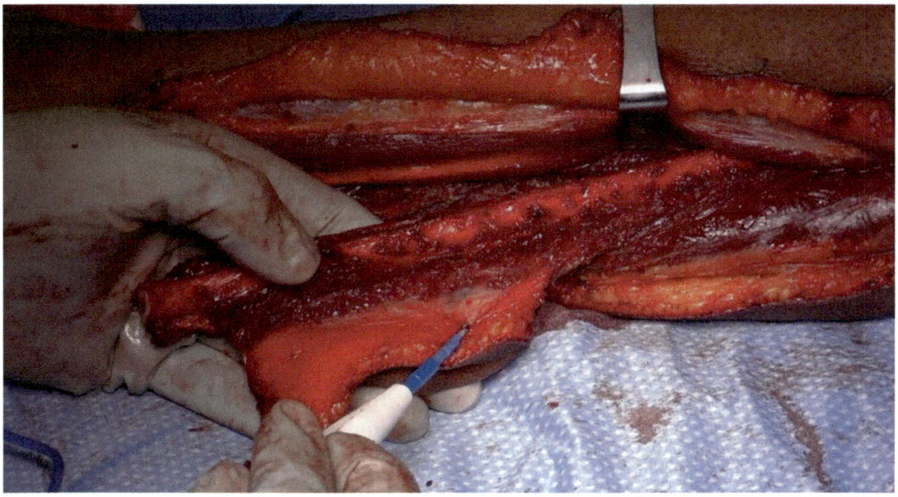

Fig. 1.8 Final mobilization of the fibula flap. The Bovie cautery tip is near the skin paddle perforator. Also note a 1–2 mm muscular cuff is preserved around the bone and pedicle

muscle. These perforators can be used to incorporate a portion of muscle into the flap in order to create a chimeric flap with skin, bone, and muscle.

The flap will be nearly completely dissected at this point (Fig. 1.8). The pedicle can be carefully freed from surrounding soft tissues in order to prepare it for microvascular anastomosis. The tibioperoneal trunk will be identified and the peroneal artery should be exposed as far proximally as possible. If cutting guides are planned, the amount of bone can be confirmed and the remaining extra bone can be stripped of periosteal attachments which will have the effect of further lengthening and exposing the pedicle.

At this point the flap should be completely mobilized. The tourniquet should be let down and the flap inspected for endosteal bleeding and pulsation within the pedicle. Occasionally, the pedicle will be cold and the pulsation within it will seem weak. It is best to soak it with papaverine and cover it with warm laps and allow it to warm up before further contouring the flap.

Mandible Reconstruction

The free vascularized osseous or osteocutaneous flap is the workhorse flap for mandible reconstruction. Several important features of the fibula flap make it a primary staple for these cases. The length of the fibula bone lends itself well to reconstructing large bony defects, which may involve three or more segments. The fibula is usually thick enough for stable dental implant placement for subsequent oral rehabilitation. The skin of the lower leg is usually thin enough to allow for closure of intraoral defects without introducing too much bulk, including buccal mucosa, alveolar coverage, floor of mouth, palate, and tongue. As long as the vascular pedicle is dissected proximally toward the takeoff from the tibio-peroneal junction, there is usually sufficient pedicle length to reach either neck for microvascular anastomosis.

There are a few key considerations in mandible reconstruction depending on the location of the anatomic defect. See below for a few tips.

Reconstructing the mandibular *symphysis* is important for appearance and for function. If a symphyseal defect is not reconstructed, then patients will have a deficient-appearing mandible due to loss of bony projection of the chin. Patients will also drool due to loss of lower lip support. Finally, patients will be dependent on a tracheostomy; without a symphysis, the hyoid bone will not be suspended to stable tissue, thus resulting in the collapse of the airway. Thus, bony reconstruction of the symphysis is recommended, when able. In our experience, it is rare for only the symphysis to be resected. More commonly, the symphysis, parasymphysis, and part of the anterior mandibular body are resected. This requires a three-segment fibular reconstruction, typically with an intraoral skin paddle. As discussed, the minimum length of the fibular segments should be 2 cm. Longer fibular segments will preserve perfusion of these segments. Once the bone is fixated to the native mandible, the hyoid bone may be resuspended to the plate of the new symphysis using 0-Prolene suture, thus facilitating decannulation of the tracheostomy in the future.

Mandible defects that involve the *condyle* can pose a reconstructive challenge. Soft-tissue flaps of posterior mandible defects are suboptimal to bony reconstructions. Multiple studies support bony reconstruction of posterior mandible defects instead of soft tissue only, pointing to better dental occlusion, function, and appearance-related outcomes [34–39]. Typically, a two-piece fibular reconstruction is necessary for a condyle/ramus segment and an angle/body segment. As discussed, the distal part of the flap should serve as the condylar reconstruction, so that the vascular pedicle comes off the mandibular body reconstruction. This fibular orientation avoids the need for a very long pedicle and minimizes the kinking of the vessels that is at risk if the proximal portion of the fibula is used for condyle reconstruction. The fibular bone can be contoured to the size and shape of the native condyle, which can be planned preoperatively using virtual surgical planning. A patient-specific prefabricated cutting guide may be used to guide precise contouring of the neocondyle. It is important to seat the neocondyle in the glenoid fossa. The capsule attachments are disrupted in the ablative part of the procedure, which results in instability and subluxation of the fibula out of the glenoid fossa. Thus, we find it helpful to suspend the neocondyle to the capsule of the glenoid fossa using a 0-Prolene suture to prevent subluxation and preserve proper occlusion. We often will place the patient in maxillomandibular fixation, followed by guiding elastics to help reestablish and maintain premorbid occlusion.

Composite defects of the mandible, which include oral mucosa, mandible bone, and external skin, can also pose a reconstructive challenge. The fibula flap can be harvested as a chimera, using two separate skin paddles on adjacent perforators for intraoral lining and external coverage and a vascularized segment of soleus muscle

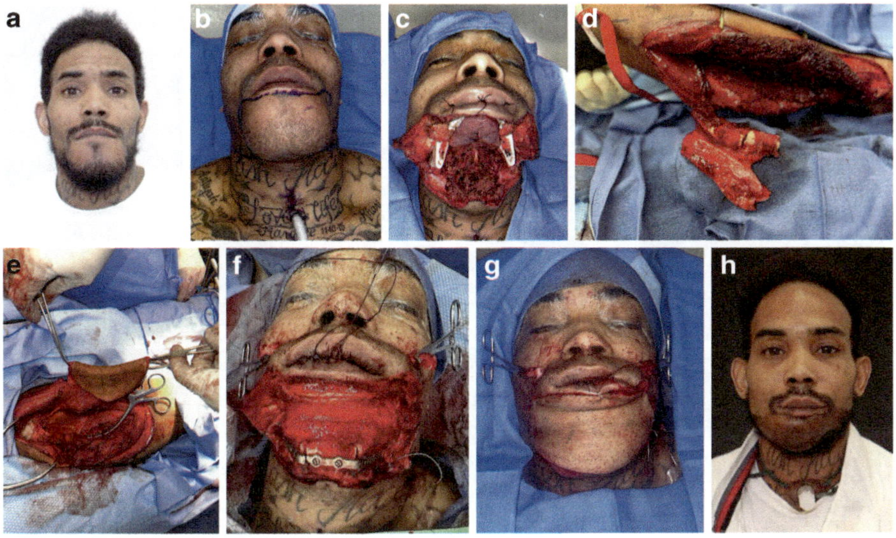

Fig. 1.9 (**a**) Preoperative view of a patient with a central mandibular osteosarcoma with skin involvement. (**b**) Preoperative soft tissue resection margins. (**c**) Composite mandibular defect. (**d**) Elevated fibula free flap prior to transfer. (**e**) Anterolateral thigh free flap with fascia lata sling for lip suspension. (**f**) Fibula flap inset. (**g**) Anterolateral thigh flap inset. (**h**) Postoperative view at 6 months

for dead space obliteration. However, the fibula donor site may not provide enough soft tissue bulk in some composite defects. Instead of a chimeric fibular flap, a second free or pedicled flap may be necessary to achieve the reconstructive goals and provide wound closure in situations where more soft tissue bulk and/or an additional skin paddle is needed. In Fig. 1.9 we share an example of a patient who underwent resection of the symphysis, parasymphysis, and anterior mandibular bodies, floor-of-mouth resection, and external chin resection for surgical treatment of osteosarcoma. This defect was successfully reconstructed with a three-segment osteocutaneous free fibula flap for mandible reconstruction and oral lining closure, followed by a free anterolateral thigh flap for external skin coverage.

Maxillary Reconstruction

Unreconstructed maxillary defects may impact facial appearance and function. Specifically, anterior maxillary defects result in poor upper lip and nasal base support, resulting in oral incompetence and nasal deformity, respectively. Palatal defects may impede oral intake of food and result in hyponasal speech, thus affecting patient quality of life. Posterior palatal defects may be closed with soft tissue only. However, in patients with anterior defects and those with total or subtotal maxillectomy, bony reconstruction in addition to soft tissue closure can provide soft

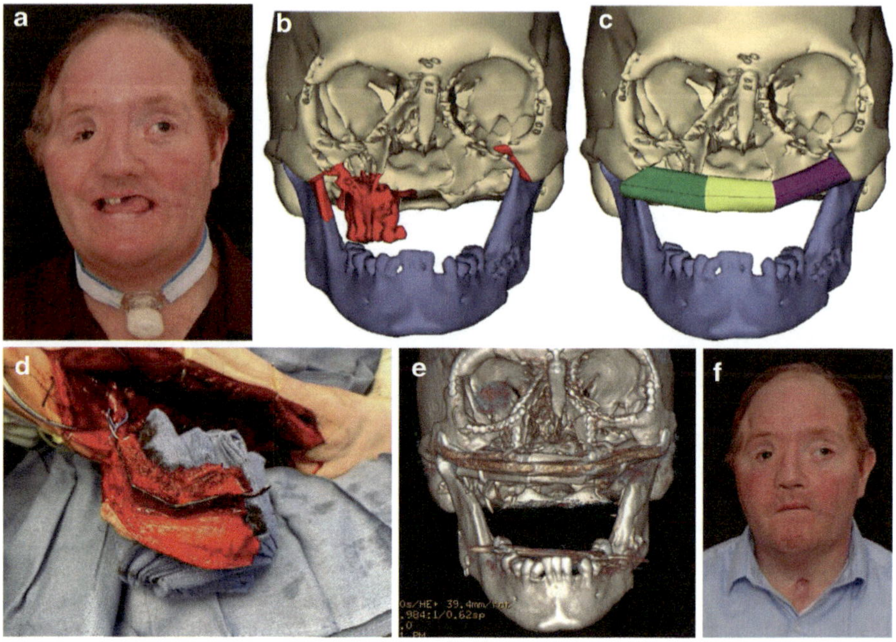

Fig. 1.10 (**a**) Preoperative view of patient with traumatic maxillary defect. (**b**) VSP images of maxillectomy defect. (**c**) VSP images of mockup of planned fibula free flap reconstruction. (**d**) Fibula free flap elevated. (**e**) Postoperative CT scan showing fibula flap in place. (**f**) Postoperative view of patient

tissue support and the opportunity for dental rehabilitation with dental implants. In Fig. 1.10 we present a case of a patient with traumatic loss of the maxilla, requiring maxillary alveolus and palatal reconstruction with a three-piece fibula flap.

Pediatric Head and Neck Reconstructions

Pediatric patients may need to undergo bony reconstruction of the maxilla or mandible in cases of benign or malignant pathology. The same principles of reconstruction apply in pediatric patients as they do for adults, with a few additional considerations. In contrast to adults, pediatric patients are growing. Thus, unreconstructed defects of the maxilla or mandible may result in progressive facial and occlusal deformity, which can be functionally and aesthetically devastating. Thus, it is important to consider bone reconstruction to minimize the deformity and functional deficit in pediatric patients. Pediatric patients will have similar anatomy to adults, but on a smaller scale. Thus, the fibular bone will be shorter and thinner, depending on the child's age, and the vascular pedicle will be shorter with smaller vessels than for adults. In addition, the periosteum that may still be adherent to the free vascular pedicle has osteogenic potential. Orthodontic treatment after reconstruction is important to reestablish and maintain normal occlusion in a patient with mixed dentition. It is necessary to monitor the growth of the fibula bone over time until skeletal maturity is reached, and dental implants may be placed for dental rehabilitation.

Extremity Long Bone Reconstruction

As mentioned previously in this chapter, the fibula flap has been used extensively in long bone reconstructions in the appendicular skeleton. Defects can be posttraumatic, oncologic, and infectious related. The fibula flap closely resembles the diameter of the radius, ulna, and clavicle (Fig. 1.11). It is slightly smaller than the humerus and will need a double-barrel construct, onlay with allograft or capanna technique (below) for femur and tibia reconstructions.

When generating an algorithm for when to use VBG for long bone reconstructions, an important factor is whether or not an articular reconstruction is required. If so, a modular endoprosthesis is preferred [40]. For articular-sparing reconstructions combinations of bone allografts and VBG are preferred for their durability and general lower complication rate, particularly in the setting of a radiated wound bed [40, 41]. Additionally, in defects greater than 6 cm and in defects requiring both bone and soft tissue flap coverage, VBG should be strongly considered [42–44].

There are three general techniques for VBG placement [40]. The first would be intercalary placement, in which the VBG is inset directly into the bone defect. The

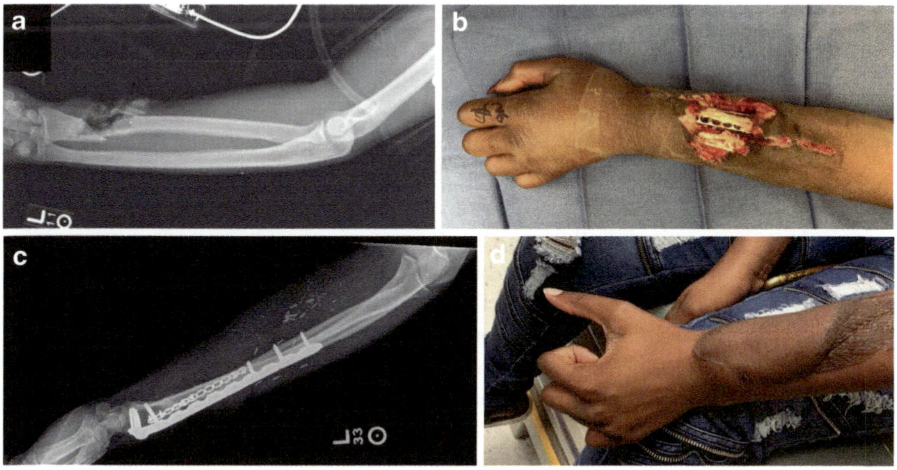

Fig. 1.11 (**a**, **b**) Ballistic injury to the distal radius with assault rifle, X-rays, and soft tissue defects. (**c**) Postoperative radiograph demonstrating intercalary placement of fibula osteocutaneous free flap. (**d**) Postop result at 2 years

second would be an onlay VBG in which an allograft is placed in the defect and the VBG is placed directly on the outer cortex of the allograft bone. This has the benefit of immediate strength and stability to the reconstruction from the allograft. The third technique would be placement of the allograft within the center of the allograft through a reamed channel (Capanna technique).

It is important to examine outcomes of these reconstructive techniques. *Mericli* et al. cited union time in oncologic defects at 14 months. Return to full weightbearing in this patient population averaged 16 months [40]. *Houdek* et al. reported union rates in 98% of patients (n = 56) with a mean time to full union of 13 months, also in the oncologic population. *Mueller* et al. looked at outcomes with pediatric patients undergoing VBG and compared union rates with onlay, Capanna, and intercalary techniques [42]. In this study, onlay and Capanna techniques had a median time to union of 13.5 and 14.6 months, respectively. Intercalary positioning had a median time to union of 3.4 months. Despite high union rates in this study (97%), reoperation occurred in 62% of lower extremity reconstructions versus 25% of upper extremity reconstructions. In the trauma patient, *Yazar* et al. reported a slightly lower union rate of 88.5% and an average time to union of 8.5 months [43]. This was a heterogeneous group of VBG, but 43 of 50 patients had a fibula free flap. These were long segment defects averaging 11.7 cm and no allograft bone was used to supplement fixation.

Capanna Technique

Capanna et al. first described an alternative technique for long bone reconstruction in which metadiaphyseal defects were reconstructed with a vascularized fibular autograft surrounded by a massive bone allograft which serves as a peripheral shell surrounding the fibula [45]. The advantages to this are that the massive allograft provides structural support while the vascularized fibula graft speeds union and revascularization of the bone allograft [46, 47]. These combined allo–/autograft reconstructions are best utilized on the long bones of the lower extremities which are the major load-bearing structures of the body. This technique has been used in the femur, tibia, and calcaneus, among other bones [45, 48–50]. Many of these defects have been quite lengthy, with Venkatramani reporting a median bone gap of 15 cm [50]. Bone union times have been reported between 5 and 24 months [16, 19–21]. Capanna published an updated account of his work in 2007 with 90 patients undergoing either tibia or femur reconstructions [18]. Lower extremity long bone defects averaged 16 cm (range 7–26 cm) and the average follow-up was 9 years. Nonunion occurred in only 10.5% of tibias and 6% of femoral reconstructions. Despite these promising results, 27.7% required at least one surgical revision.

The surgical technique is well described [18, 45, 46, 51]. The fibula graft size should be 6 cm longer than the intended bone defect, with 2–3 cm of fibula allowed to protrude as a “peg” from either end of the large bone allograft. The bone allograft should be rinsed and the cancellous bone reamed to allow precise fitting of the vascularized fibula flap down the center of the bony allograft. A cutting burr is then used to make a linear trough in the cortex of the bone allograft to allow unimpeded passage of the peroneal vascular pedicle. The fibular "pegs" are then placed in a reamed channel in the proximal and distal bone remnants with plate and screw fixation performed in standard fashion. Often a K-wire is required to be placed through the allograft/autograft construct to prevent rotation of the fibula flap within the canal of the bone allograft. A skin paddle can often be omitted but may be required in more distal reconstructions as the soft tissue envelope thins. As a reconstructive option, the Capanna technique offers an innovate way to provide immediate strength to the bony reconstruction and the benefits of a VBG.

Spine Reconstruction

The fibula flap has also developed into a useful tool for spinal reconstructions [52–55]. Generally speaking, the fibula is going to be used to reconstruct the spine following corpectomy, but can also be used for posterior column reconstruction. *Goldman* et al. have reported a successful 5-level anterior cervical fusion through a transoral approach using a vascularized fibula osseocutaneous free flap [56]. *Erdmann* et al. reported four cases of salvage reconstruction with a fibula free flap of failed anterior spine fixation with cases representing most spine levels [57]. In this series reconstruction was done with staged posterior instrumentation followed in 1 week by anterior corpectomy and fibula free flap. A trough was created in the nonaffected spinal bodies to allow for placement of either a single- or double-barrel fibula flap. Recipient vessels were lumbar arteries off the aorta and end saphenous vein grafts from the aorta to the peroneal artery to ease inset. Recipient veins utilized in these cases were lumbar and gonadal veins. All patients in this series experienced complete union and graft incorporation. Creativity is required for recipient vessel selection. In Asaad's description of thoracic fibula flap spinal reconstruction, the intercostal vessels were most commonly used for recipient vessels [54]. Notably, in this study, union time between pedicled rib and fibula free flap reconstructions of the anterior corpus was not significantly different (median 9 months in each group).

A variety of fixation techniques have been described. *Doi* et al. utilized an overlapping notch joining both the proximal and distal vertebral corpora with a stabilizing lip of bone being used to maintain position and length [52]. *Bindal* et al. described a noninstrumented technique for cervical spine fusion [53]. In this technique the patient was placed in 50 lb. of tong traction and underwent corpectomy and precise wedge fibula free flap placement and then release of traction which caused press fixation of the flap within the corpus. This is an innovative technique to avoid instrumentation in cases of osteomyelitis.

Merici published data from MD Anderson in 2022 comparing NVBG to fibula free flap for spinal reconstructions [58]. Nonunions were 41.7% (NVBG) versus 6.3% in the fibula free flap group. Neurologic complications were also much lower in the fibula group (0%) versus NVBG (25%). Again, a variety of recipient vessels were required. In particular, vein grafting was required in 18.7% of arterial and 25% of venous anastomoses. This highlights the need to be creative and prepared when performing spinal reconstructions with this flap.

Donor Site Management

Care and attention should be utilized when closing the fibula flap donor site. When closing the authors place a closed suction drain in the dead space which normally remains about a week. The muscle belly of the FHL should be reattached using absorbable suture to the remaining deep posterior compartment muscles. This is done to tension it and hopefully prevent hammertoe deformity. Distally, near the ankle, there will be deficient soft tissue. The authors will reapproximate the peroneus tendons over the cut end of the fibula to provide additional soft tissue coverage over the bone. As the closure proceeds proximally, the lateral compartment muscles will be sutured to the soleus and lateral gastrocnemius muscles to recreate the anatomy of the area. The dermis and skin are then closed in standard fashion.

If there is a skin deficit that cannot be closed primarily, typically a split thickness skin graft will be required to cover this donor site. This can be tricky as much of the paratenon will be missing and the wound bed will have a lot of exposed tendon if the deep closure is not done properly. If it appears that the wound bed will not take, a dermal substitute is probably best to prevent a prolonged course of dressing changes over an area of poor graft take.

Our final dressing consists of bulky cotton leg wraps with ace bandages for pressure relief and swelling. The patient is allowed to ambulate ad lib in compression at postoperative day #5. If there is a skin graft, the dressing is changed at postoperative day #5 and then placed in an Unna boot for a week.

Patients should be counseled that they may have lower extremity edema for several weeks and even months after surgery, but ambulation should be encouraged as this will speed recovery. Patients can also experience transitory numbness of the lateral ankle which should recover in time.

Outcomes and Complications

Successful initial flap survival is paramount when performing fibula flap reconstructions, particularly in head and neck patients. Preoperative workup and planning with medical optimization of the infirm patient cannot also be overstated. This may not be possible in the patient with newly diagnosed head and neck cancer but attempts should be made to cease tobacco and nicotine use and manage comorbidities such as hypertension and diabetes.

Intraoperatively, attempts should be made to achieve normothermia and manage hypotension and blood loss. We use underwarming blankets and also place air warmers over the contralateral leg and chest. Blood loss can be minimized with the use of a tourniquet and meticulous hemostasis. Our unit routinely transfuses blood products postoperatively to keep a hemoglobin of $\geq$7 g/dL.

At the conclusion of the case, the skin paddle must be well perfused and a watertight seal achieved intraorally. The authors' surgical team always performs a leak test intraorally before closure of the neck by filling the oral cavity with saline and inspecting for leaking into the neck wound.

Postoperatively, care should be taken to monitor the skin closures carefully. Any signs of neck erythema or drainage can be a harbinger of a salivary fistula. Oral-cutaneous fistulas can be disastrous and take months to heal. Early salivary fistulas and neck infections in the author's own experience have shown a high chance of flap vascular thrombosis and failure. Carotid blowout can occur, and in frail patients, prolonged trach and enteral feeding can be required in the event of a flap failure. The senior author has also observed a near fatal case of necrotizing soft tissue infection in the neck of a patient after an oral closure breakdown with saliva pooling in the neck. Secondary reconstructions in those patients with prior flap failure are incrementally more challenging so it is very important that the initial operation be done well and has a good outcome.

In the event of a skin paddle loss or necrosis in an intraoral location, a decision will need to be made quickly as to how to proceed. The viability of the bone component of the flap needs to be determined. Typically, during a debridement, the authors will confirm viability of the bone by signs of bleeding, handheld doppler exam on the pedicle, visualization of the pedicle, and by intraoperative laser angiography. If the entire flap is necrotic, then a new fibula flap should be done immediately. If the skin paddle only is necrotic, then the options could be as follows: primary closure if possible, pedicled tongue flap for small openings, secondary fasciocutaneous free flap (e.g., radial forearm free flap), or locoregional flap such as the pectoralis major musculocutaneous flap.

In the truly septic head and neck patient with flap loss, the entire flap and hardware will need to be debrided for source control, wide drainage placed, and an external fixator placed to maintain mandibular continuity and soft tissue relationships if possible. Delayed reconstruction can be planned 6–12 months later after the wound bed has matured and the patient's weight and nutritional status have been optimized.

Long-term goals of reconstruction with vascularized fibula flaps should be bone union at the recipient site, no bone infections or nonunions, healing of the donor site, and return of normal ambulation. Our postop imaging protocol consists of plain films prior to discharge for extremity and trunk flaps. For head and neck patients we get a postop day #7 ct of the head and neck with 3D reconstructions. Serial films are done at 3 months, 6 months, and 9 months and then as indicated until radiographic evidence of bony union occurs. This is particularly important as there can be sites of nonunions that need to be monitored and potentially bone grafted again. Loosening and fracturing of hardware can also occur and should be monitored.

Conclusions

The fibula free flap is truly a workhorse flap that every plastic surgeon should be familiar with. New technological improvements are rapidly expanding the precision and speed of flap elevation. The flap can be used in a variety of scenarios for bone and soft tissue reconstruction including head and neck, extremity long bone, spine, and pelvis. Complications can occur but generally total flap loss should be low single digits and the donor site allows for a return to normal ambulation in most patients.

References

1. Taylor GI, Miller GD, Ham FJ. The free vascularized bone graft. A clinical extension of microvascular techniques. Plast Reconstr Surg. 1975;55(5):533–44. https://doi.org/10.1097/00006534-197505000-00002.
2. Hidalgo DA. Fibula free flap: a new method of mandible reconstruction. Plast Reconstr Surg. 1989;84(1):71–9.
3. Cordeiro PG, Disa JJ, Hidalgo DA, Hu QY. Reconstruction of the mandible with osseous free flaps: a 10-year experience with 150 consecutive patients. Plast Reconstr Surg. 1999;104(5):1314–20. https://doi.org/10.1097/00006534-199910000-00011.
4. Zlotolow IM, Huryn JM, Piro JD, Lenchewski E, Hidalgo DA. Osseointegrated implants and functional prosthetic rehabilitation in microvascular fibula free flap reconstructed mandibles. Am J Surg. 1992;164(6):677–81. https://doi.org/10.1016/s0002-9610(05)80733-0.
5. Hidalgo DA. Fibula free flap mandibular reconstruction. Clin Plast Surg. 1994;21(1):25–35.
6. Hidalgo DA, Rekow A. A review of 60 consecutive fibula free flap mandible reconstructions. Plast Reconstr Surg. 1995;96(3):585–96; discussion 597–602.
7. Hidalgo DA. Fibula free flap mandible reconstruction. Microsurgery. 1994;15(4):238–44. https://doi.org/10.1002/micr.1920150404.
8. Wei FC, Seah CS, Tsai YC, Liu SJ, Tsai MS. Fibula osteoseptocutaneous flap for reconstruction of composite mandibular defects. Plast Reconstr Surg. 1994;93(2):294–304; discussion 305-6.
9. Wei FC, Chuang SS, Yim KK. The sensate fibula osteoseptocutaneous flap: a preliminary report. Br J Plast Surg. 1994;47(8):544–7. https://doi.org/10.1016/0007-1226(94)90137-6.
10. Yim KK, Wei FC. Fibula osteoseptocutaneous flap for mandible reconstruction. Microsurgery. 1994;15(4):245–9. https://doi.org/10.1002/micr.1920150405.
11. Wei FC, Santamaria E, Chang YM, Chen HC. Mandibular reconstruction with fibular osteoseptocutaneous free flap and simultaneous placement of osseointegrated dental implants. J Craniofac Surg. 1997;8(6):512–21. https://doi.org/10.1097/00001665-199711000-00018.
12. Santamaria E, Wei FC, Chen HC. Fibula osteoseptocutaneous flap for reconstruction of osteoradionecrosis of the mandible. Plast Reconstr Surg. 1998;101(4):921–9. https://doi.org/10.1097/00006534-199804040-00006.
13. Wei FC, Demirkan F, Chen HC, Chen IH. Double free flaps in reconstruction of extensive composite mandibular defects in head and neck cancer. Plast Reconstr Surg. 1999;103(1):39–47. https://doi.org/10.1097/00006534-199901000-00008.
14. Hsieh CH, Jeng SF, Chen SH, Wei FC. Folded free vascularized fibular grafts for the reconstruction of combined segmental bone defects of distal tibia and fibula. J Trauma. 2004;56(2):437–9. https://doi.org/10.1097/01.TA.0000023167.68453.9C.
15. Chana JS, Chang YM, Wei FC, et al. Segmental mandibulectomy and immediate free fibula osteoseptocutaneous flap reconstruction with endosteal implants: an ideal treatment

method for mandibular ameloblastoma. Plast Reconstr Surg. 2004;113(1):80–7. https://doi.org/10.1097/01.PRS.0000097719.69616.29.
16. Foster RD, Anthony JP, Sharma A, Pogrel MA. Vascularized bone flaps versus nonvascularized bone grafts for mandibular reconstruction: an outcome analysis of primary bony union and endosseous implant success. Head Neck. 1999;21(1):66–71. https://doi.org/10.1002/(sici)1097-0347(199901)21:1<66::aid-hed9>3.0.co;2-z.
17. Pogrel MA, Podlesh S, Anthony JP, Alexander J. A comparison of vascularized and nonvascularized bone grafts for reconstruction of mandibular continuity defects. J Oral Maxillofac Surg. 1997;55(11):1200–6. https://doi.org/10.1016/s0278-2391(97)90165-8.
18. Capanna R, Campanacci DA, Belot N, et al. A new reconstructive technique for intercalary defects of long bones: the association of massive allograft with vascularized fibular autograft. Long-term results and comparison with alternative techniques. Orthop Clin North Am. 2007;38(1):51–60, vi. https://doi.org/10.1016/j.ocl.2006.10.008.
19. Taylor GI, Corlett RJ, Ashton MW. The evolution of free vascularized bone transfer: a 40-year experience. Plast Reconstr Surg. 2016;137(4):1292–305. https://doi.org/10.1097/PRS.0000000000002040.
20. Mathes SJ, Nahai F. Classification of the vascular anatomy of muscles: experimental and clinical correlation. Plast Reconstr Surg. 1981;67(2):177–87.
21. Mathes S, Nahai F. Reconstructive surgery: principles, anatomy, and technique, vol. 2. Quality Medical Publishing, Inc.; 1997.
22. Taylor GI, Wilson KR, Rees MD, Corlett RJ, Cole WG. The anterior tibial vessels and their role in epiphyseal and diaphyseal transfer of the fibula: experimental study and clinical applications. Br J Plast Surg. 1988;41(5):451–69. https://doi.org/10.1016/0007-1226(88)90001-x.
23. Wei FC, Chen HC, Chuang CC, Noordhoff MS. Fibular osteoseptocutaneous flap: anatomic study and clinical application. Plast Reconstr Surg. 1986;78(2):191–200. https://doi.org/10.1097/00006534-198608000-00008.
24. Netter FH. Atlas of human anatomy. Novartis; 1997.
25. Gholami M, Hedjazi A, Kiamarz MA. Evaluation of anatomic variations of fibula free flap in human fresh cadavers. World J Plast Surg. 2019;8(2):229–36. https://doi.org/10.29252/wjps.8.2.229.
26. Kocabiyik N, Yalçin B, Ozan H. Variations of the nutrient artery of the fibula. Clin Anat. 2007;20(4):440–3. https://doi.org/10.1002/ca.20442.
27. Ni Y, Zhang X, Zhang Z, et al. Assessment of fibula flap with flexor hallucis longus's effect on head & neck tumor patients' quality of life and function of donor site. Oral Oncol. 2020;100:104489. https://doi.org/10.1016/j.oraloncology.2019.104489.
28. Yu P, Chang EI, Hanasono MM. Design of a reliable skin paddle for the fibula osteocutaneous flap: perforator anatomy revisited. Plast Reconstr Surg. 2011;128(2):440–6. https://doi.org/10.1097/PRS.0b013e31821e7058.
29. Benedict KC, Horriat NL, McIntyre BC. Free fibula flap mandibular reconstruction: a video demonstrating operative technique. Plast Reconstr Surg Glob Open. 2023;11(11):e5380. https://doi.org/10.1097/GOX.0000000000005380.
30. Pucci R, Weyh A, Smotherman C, Valentini V, Bunnell A, Fernandes R. Accuracy of virtual planned surgery versus conventional free-hand surgery for reconstruction of the mandible with osteocutaneous free flaps. Int J Oral Maxillofac Surg. 2020;49(9):1153–61. https://doi.org/10.1016/j.ijom.2020.02.018.
31. Tang NSJ, Ahmadi I, Ramakrishnan A. Virtual surgical planning in fibula free flap head and neck reconstruction: a systematic review and meta-analysis. J Plast Reconstr Aesthet Surg. 2019;72(9):1465–77. https://doi.org/10.1016/j.bjps.2019.06.013.
32. Mazzola F, Smithers F, Cheng K, et al. Time and cost-analysis of virtual surgical planning for head and neck reconstruction: a matched pair analysis. Oral Oncol. 2020;100:104491. https://doi.org/10.1016/j.oraloncology.2019.104491.
33. Kurlander DE, Garvey PB, Largo RD, et al. The cost utility of virtual surgical planning and computer-assisted design/computer-assisted manufacturing in mandible reconstruction using

the free fibula osteocutaneous flap. J Reconstr Microsurg. 2023;39(3):221–30. https://doi.org/10.1055/s-0042-1755260.
34. Cohen Z, Zhang KK, Kim M, et al. A preliminary analysis of patient reported outcomes following posterolateral mandible reconstruction: the role of flap type. J Surg Oncol. 2024;129(3):617–28. https://doi.org/10.1002/jso.27520.
35. Hanasono MM, Zevallos JP, Skoracki RJ, Yu P. A prospective analysis of bony versus soft-tissue reconstruction for posterior mandibular defects. Plast Reconstr Surg. 2010;125(5):1413–21. https://doi.org/10.1097/PRS.0b013e3181d62aef.
36. Mosahebi A, Chaudhry A, McCarthy CM, et al. Reconstruction of extensive composite posterolateral mandibular defects using nonosseous free tissue transfer. Plast Reconstr Surg. 2009;124(5):1571–7. https://doi.org/10.1097/PRS.0b013e3181b98b78.
37. King TW, Gallas MT, Robb GL, Lalani Z, Miller MJ. Aesthetic and functional outcomes using osseous or soft-tissue free flaps. J Reconstr Microsurg. 2002;18(5):365–71. https://doi.org/10.1055/s-2002-33017.
38. Mizukami T, Hyodo I, Fukamizu H, Mineta H. Reconstruction of lateral mandibular defect: a comparison of functional and aesthetic outcomes of bony reconstruction vs soft tissue reconstruction – long-term follow-up. Acta Otolaryngol. 2013;133(12):1304–10. https://doi.org/10.3109/00016489.2013.824111.
39. Dimovska EOF, Clibbon J, Heaton M, Viswanathan N, Ridha H, James R. Challenging the orthodoxy of mandibular reconstructions comparing functional outcomes in osseous versus soft tissue reconstructions of the posterolateral mandible. J Reconstr Microsurg. 2020;36(1):21–7. https://doi.org/10.1055/s-0039-1694044.
40. Mericli AF, Asaad M, Lewis VO, et al. Free fibula flap for extremity oncologic defects: factors influencing union and functional outcomes. Plast Reconstr Surg. 2023;151(4):885–96. https://doi.org/10.1097/PRS.0000000000010014.
41. Houdek MT, Wagner ER, Bishop AT, et al. Complications and long-term outcomes of free fibula reconstruction following resection of a malignant tumor in the extremities. Plast Reconstr Surg. 2017;139(2):510e–9e. https://doi.org/10.1097/PRS.0000000000003004.
42. Mueller MA, Mericli AF, Roubaud MS, et al. Comparing fibula flap insetting techniques for pediatric oncologic extremity reconstruction. Plast Reconstr Surg. 2024;153(3):636e–43e. https://doi.org/10.1097/PRS.0000000000010613.
43. Yazar S, Lin CH, Wei FC. One-stage reconstruction of composite bone and soft-tissue defects in traumatic lower extremities. Plast Reconstr Surg. 2004;114(6):1457–66. https://doi.org/10.1097/01.prs.0000138811.88807.65.
44. Zhen P, Hu YY, Luo ZJ, Liu XY, Lu H, Li XS. One-stage treatment and reconstruction of gustilo type III open tibial shaft fractures with a vascularized fibular osteoseptocutaneous flap graft. J Orthop Trauma. 2010;24(12):745–51. https://doi.org/10.1097/BOT.0b013e3181d88a07.
45. Capanna R, Bufalini C, Campanacci M. A new technique for reconstructions of large metadiaphyseal bone defects. Orthop Traumatol. 1993;2(3):159–77.
46. Moran SL, Shin AY, Bishop AT. The use of massive bone allograft with intramedullary free fibular flap for limb salvage in a pediatric and adolescent population. Plast Reconstr Surg. 2006;118(2):413–9. https://doi.org/10.1097/01.prs.0000227682.71527.2b.
47. Houdek MT, Wagner ER, Stans AA, et al. What is the outcome of allograft and intramedullary free fibula (Capanna technique) in pediatric and adolescent patients with bone tumors? Clin Orthop Relat Res. 2016;474(3):660–8. https://doi.org/10.1007/s11999-015-4204-2.
48. Hamrouni N, Højvig JH, Petersen MM, Hettwer W, Jensen LT, Bonde CT. Total calcaneal reconstruction using a massive bone allograft and a distally pedicled osteocutaneous fibula flap: a novel technique to prevent amputation after calcaneal malignancy. J Plast Reconstr Aesthet Surg. 2023;76:44–8. https://doi.org/10.1016/j.bjps.2022.10.039.
49. Rajasekaran RB, Jayaramaraju D, Venkataramani H, Agraharam D, Shanmuganathan RS, Shanmuganathan R. Successful reconstruction of a post-traumatic defect of 16 cm of the distal femur by modified Capanna's technique (vascularised free fibula combined with allograft) – a

case report and technical note. Trauma Case Rep. 2018;17:29–32. https://doi.org/10.1016/j.tcr.2018.09.007.
50. Venkatramani H, Sabapathy SR, Dheenadayalan J, Devendra A, Rajasekaran S. Reconstruction of post-traumatic long segment bone defects of the lower end of the femur by free vascularized fibula combined with allograft (modified Capanna's technique). Eur J Trauma Emerg Surg. 2015;41(1):17–24. https://doi.org/10.1007/s00068-014-0451-2.
51. Bakri K, Stans AA, Mardini S, Moran SL. Combined massive allograft and intramedullary vascularized fibula transfer: the capanna technique for lower-limb reconstruction. Semin Plast Surg. 2008;22(3):234–41. https://doi.org/10.1055/s-2008-1081406.
52. Doi K, Kawai S, Sumiura S, Sakai K. Anterior cervical fusion using the free vascularized fibular graft. Spine (Phila Pa 1976). 1988;13(11):1239–44. https://doi.org/10.1097/00007632-198811000-00006.
53. Bindal S, Fairchild B, Lamaris GA, Cochran JA. Noninstrumented free fibula flap for cervical osteomyelitis. Oper Neurosurg (Hagerstown). 2023; https://doi.org/10.1227/ons.0000000000001019.
54. Asaad M, Houdek MT, Huang TCT, Rose PS, Moran SL. Vascularized bone flap options for complex thoracic spinal reconstruction. Plast Reconstr Surg. 2022;149(3):515e–25e. https://doi.org/10.1097/PRS.0000000000008837.
55. McChesney GR, Mericli AF, Rhines LD, Bird JE. The future of free vascularized fibular grafts in oncologic spinal and pelvic reconstruction. J Spine Surg. 2019;5(2):291–5. https://doi.org/10.21037/jss.2019.04.01.
56. Goldman JJ, Huynh KA, Elfallal W, Chaiyasate K, Fahim DK. Cervical spine and craniocervical junction reconstruction with a vascularized fibula free flap. World Neurosurg. 2020;144:34–8. https://doi.org/10.1016/j.wneu.2020.08.057.
57. Erdmann D, Meade RA, Lins RE, McCann RL, Richardson WJ, Levin LS. Use of the microvascular free fibula transfer as a salvage reconstruction for failed anterior spine surgery due to chronic osteomyelitis. Plast Reconstr Surg. 2006;117(7):2438–45; discussion 2446-7. https://doi.org/10.1097/01.prs.0000219077.73229.af.
58. Mericli AF, Boukovalas S, Rhines LD, Adelman DM, Hanasono MM, Chang EI. Free fibula flap for restoration of spinal stability after oncologic vertebrectomy is predictive of bony union. Plast Reconstr Surg. 2020;145(1):219–29. https://doi.org/10.1097/PRS.0000000000006382.

Chapter 2
Fibula Flap with Physis

Mohamed Morsy, Rou Wan, and Steven L. Moran

Introduction

Bony defects involving the physis in skeletally immature subjects are very challenging problems to reconstruct. These can be congenital, posttraumatic, postinfection, and post tumor excision. A complex reconstruction is needed for these defects which will often require multiple components to reconstruct including the bony defect, growing physis, articulating surface, and supporting ligaments [1–5].

Transferring nonvascularized growth plates has been attempted as early as the end of the nineteenth century experimentally and clinically [6]. The first successful report was in 1924 which was followed by a number of similar nonvascularized transfers with highly variable results [7].

Vascularized proximal fibular transfer was first reported by Pho in 1979, where he transferred the proximal fibula in an adult to reconstruct the distal radius [8]. This transfer did not contain a growth plate. In the same year, Weiland et al. reported the first two cases of vascularized growth plate transfers [9].

Earlier, proximal fibular epiphyseal transfer utilized the peroneal vessels as the pedicle. The peroneal vessels were concluded to be insufficient to support the physis due to disappointing results [10]. Bipedicled transfers were attempted adding either the anterior tibial vessels or the inferior lateral genicular vessels to support the physis. This modification produced better outcomes but was more technically

M. Morsy
Department of Orthopaedic Surgery, The University of Alabama at Birmingham, Birmingham, AL, USA

Department of Orthopaedic Surgery, Assiut University Faculty of Medicine, Assiut University, Assiut, Egypt

R. Wan · S. L. Moran (✉)
Division of Plastic Surgery, Mayo Clinic, Rochester, MN, USA
e-mail: Moran.Steven@mayo.edu

J. P. Agarwal, D. W. Mathes (eds.), *Bone Flaps in Reconstructive Surgery*,
https://doi.org/10.1007/978-3-032-12540-8_2

demanding and had a higher complication risk [11, 12]. Taylor et al. conducted a cadaveric study confirming the role of the anterior tibial vessels in providing blood supply to the proximal fibula and was the first to report on the successful clinical use of the anterior tibial vessels as a single pedicle [10]. Later on, Innocenti et al. described the "reverse flow" technique to harvest the proximal fibula on the anterior tibial vessels as a single pedicle. This allowed for a longer pedicle as well as the ability to harvest variable lengths of the fibular shaft as needed [13, 14]. Having to meticulously dissect the deep peroneal nerve and its branches in addition to the occasional need to divide and repair some of these during the harvest is a major drawback [15]. More recently, Yang et al. reported using the inferior lateral genicular vessels as a single vesicle and a small case series [16].

This chapter discusses the most recent anatomical description of the vascularity of the proximal fibula for safe harvest as well as the standard harvest technique.

Indications

Proximal fibular epiphyseal transfer is indicated in bony defects in skeletally immature patients involving the loss of the growing physis for virtually any long bone. As for anatomical locations, this can include but is not limited to:

- The distal radius.
- The proximal humerus.
- The proximal femur.
- The distal ulna.
- The distal femoral condyle.

Anatomy

Flap Components

This flap is composed of the proximal fibula including the fibular physis and epiphysis with an adjacent length of the fibular metaphysis and diaphysis. The flap includes the articular surface of the proximal tibiofibular joint as well as variable length from the biceps tendon as needed.

Vascular Supply

The standard harvest technique for this flap utilizes the anterior tibial vessels as the pedicle. The anterior tibial vessels are harvested distally, preserving the branches going to the head of the fibula and then variable length can be harvested from the vessels as needed.

Previous anatomical studies that were done on the blood supply of the fibular head pointed out the importance of the "artery of the fibular neck" as the main supplying branch. That said, there was great variability in the anatomical description of this branch [10, 17–19]. Innocenti et al. based their flap on the anterior tibial artery and a branch coming out from it, which they named the "recurrent epiphyseal artery." They were able to view it in the preoperative angiograms as well as in their intraoperative dissection [13].

In a more recent detailed anatomical study, the vascularity of the proximal fibula was studied using injection techniques, anatomical dissections, and high-resolution CT angiography [4]. This study showed the presence of a consistent rich anastomotic network supplying the head of the fibula. Six vessels were identified contributing to this network. These were the inferior lateral genicular artery (ILGA), the circumflex fibular artery (CFA), the posterior tibial recurrent artery (PTRA), the first recurrent epiphyseal artery (FREA), the second recurrent epiphyseal artery (SREA), and the superficial peroneal artery (SPA). These all originated from either the popliteal artery, the tibioperoneal trunk, or the anterior tibial artery (Figs. 2.1 and 2.2). Of prime importance for the purpose of harvesting the flap are the first and the second recurrent epiphyseal arteries. The FREA originates from either the anterior tibial artery directly or the anterior tibial recurrent artery (ATRA), which in turn originates from the anterior tibial artery. The SREA originates exclusively from the ATRA (Fig. 2.3). We believe that both of these arteries can support the flap, although

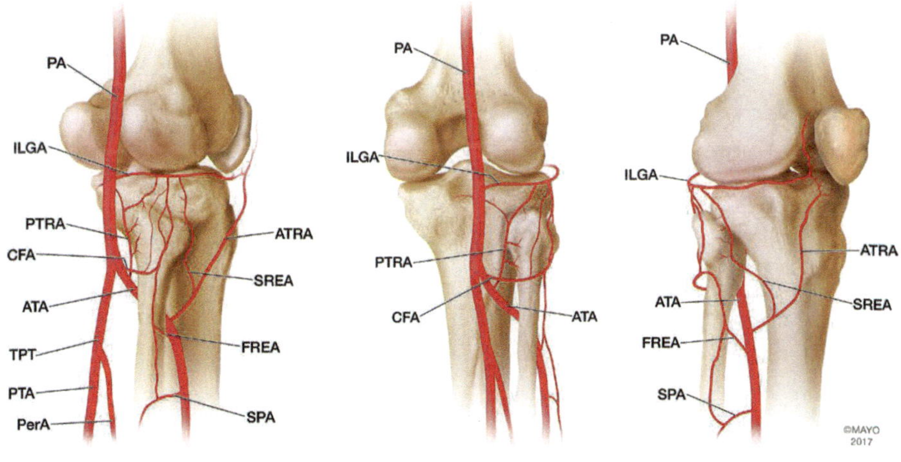

Fig. 2.1 The most commonly occurring vascular pattern supplying the fibular head is shown in the illustration with three perspectives: posterolateral (*left*), posterior (*center*), and anterolateral (*right*). *PA* popliteal artery, *ATA* anterior tibial artery, *TPT* tibio-peroneal trunk, *PTA* posterior tibial artery, *PerA* peroneal artery, *ILGA* inferior lateral genicular artery, *CFA* circumflex fibular artery, *PTRA* posterior tibial recurrent artery, *ATRA* anterior tibial recurrent artery, *FREA* first recurrent epiphyseal artery, *SREA* second recurrent epiphyseal artery, *SPA* superficial peroneal artery. (Reprinted with permission from Mayo Foundation for Medical Education and Research. All rights reserved)

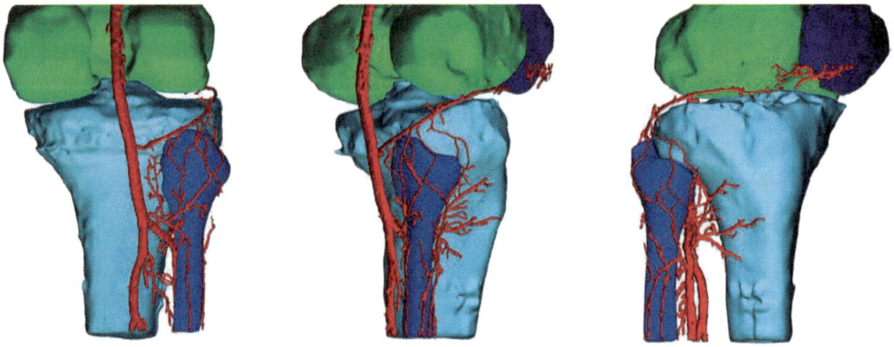

Fig. 2.2 Three-dimensional reconstruction from a high-resolution computed tomographic scan of a specimen revealed the most common vascular pattern supplying the fibular head. A pattern similar to this for the inferior lateral genicular artery was present in 96% of specimens, in 36% for the circumflex fibular artery, in 79% for the posterior tibial recurrent artery, in 57% for the first recurrent epiphyseal artery, and in 100% for both the second recurrent epiphyseal artery and the superficial peroneal artery. Views from posterior (*left*), posterolateral (*center*), and anterolateral (*right*) are displayed. (Copyright © 2018 by the American Society of Plastic Surgeons. Reprinted with permission from Morsy et al. [4]. All rights reserved)

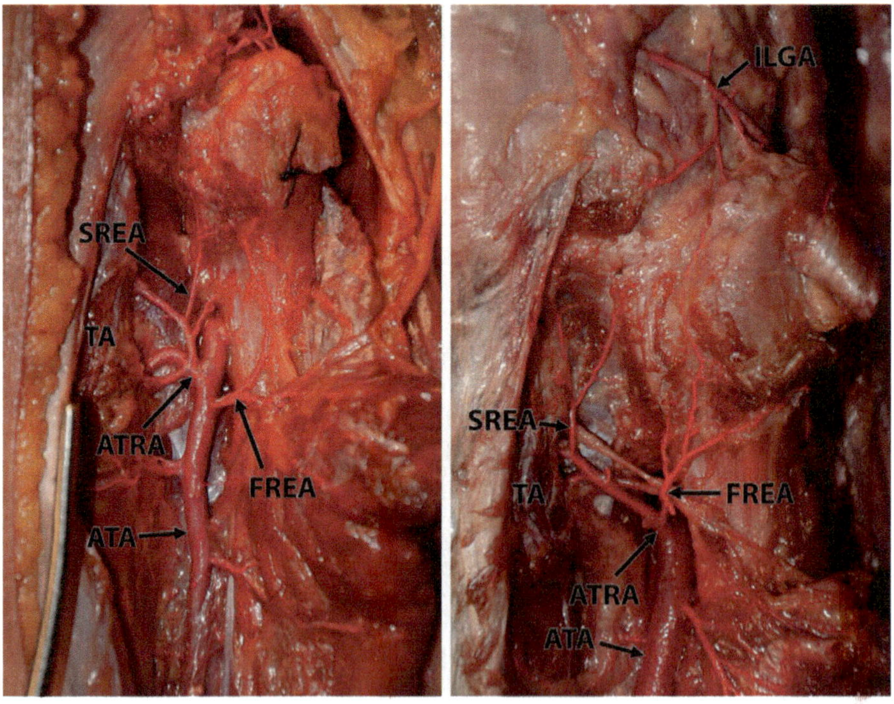

Fig. 2.3 The origin, course, and branches of the first and second recurrent epiphyseal arteries are illustrated in two specimens. The two variations are shown with the first recurrent epiphyseal artery arising from the anterior tibial recurrent artery (*left*) and from the anterior tibial recurrent artery (*right*). *ATA* anterior tibial artery, *ATRA* anterior tibial recurrent artery, *FREA* first recurrent epiphyseal artery, *SREA* second recurrent epiphyseal artery, *TA* tibialis anterior muscle. (Copyright © 2018 by the American Society of Plastic Surgeons. Reprinted with permission from Morsy et al. [4]. All rights reserved.)

the FREA has a larger caliber and is probably more favorable. During harvest of the flap, it is advised against dissection of the individual FREA or SREA. They are usually harvested within the muscle cuff surrounding the head and neck to prevent injury to the delicate vessels, which may compromise flap vascularity. The only time to do such a tedious dissection is in the instance of dissecting or salvaging one of the major motor branches of the deep peroneal nerve. The ILGA can also support the flap but is disadvantaged by the smaller caliber and short length as compared to the anterior tibial artery when used as a pedicle (Fig. 2.4).

The anterior tibial artery can support the proximal two-thirds of the fibular shaft to be included with the flap [10]. The fibular shaft receives multiple periosteal branches from the anterior tibial artery as it runs distally. These small branches run laterally anterior to the interosseous membrane and preserving these is crucial for maintaining vascularity to the shaft [14].

Another important anatomical point is the relationship of the motor branches of the deep peroneal nerve to the anterior tibial vessels and their branches supplying the head of the fibula. In the region of the proximal fibula, the deep peroneal nerve gives 2–4 motor branches to the tibialis anterior muscle that have a variable relationship to the recurrent epiphyseal vessels. The FREA had at least 1 motor branch running deep to it and the SREA was less likely to have a motor branch

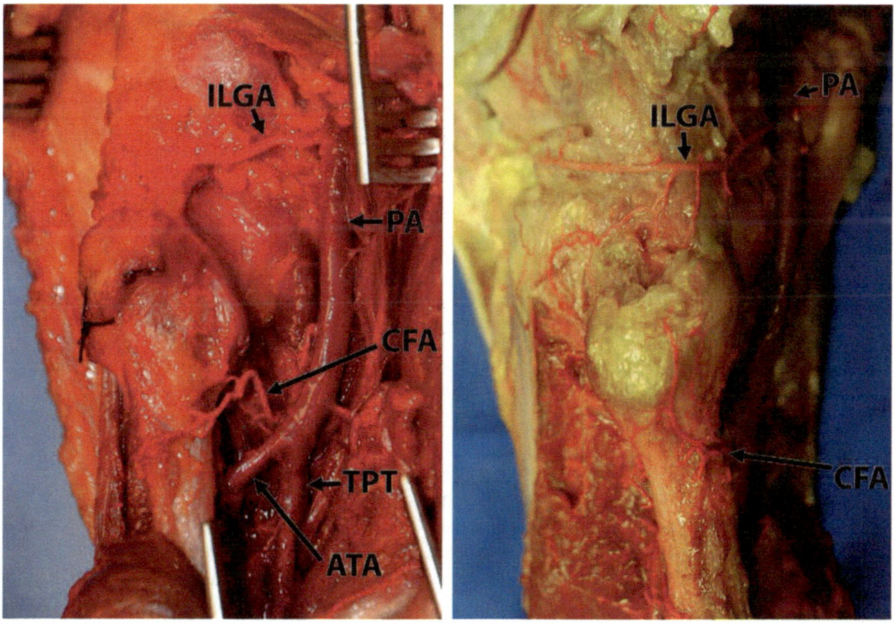

Fig. 2.4 The origin, course, and branches of the inferior lateral genicular artery supplying the fibular head are shown in two specimens. *PA* popliteal artery, *ATA* anterior tibial artery, *TPT* tibioperoneal trunk, *ILGA* inferior lateral genicular artery, *CFA* circumflex fibular artery. (Copyright © 2018 by the American Society of Plastic Surgeons. Reprinted with permission from Morsy et al. [4]. All rights reserved)

running deep to it. Distally, the deep peroneal nerve can also have motor branches running deep to the vessels or running in between the components of the pedicle. In such cases mentioned above, meticulous dissection of the nerves has to be undertaken, and in certain instances, a nerve branch may have to be divided and sutured back together (Figs. 2.5, 2.6, and 2.7). Transient foot drop is a common complication that recovers within 3–6 months, which has been reported in up to 25% or even higher [5, 11, 15]. Permanent tibialis anterior paralysis was reported in one patient [11].

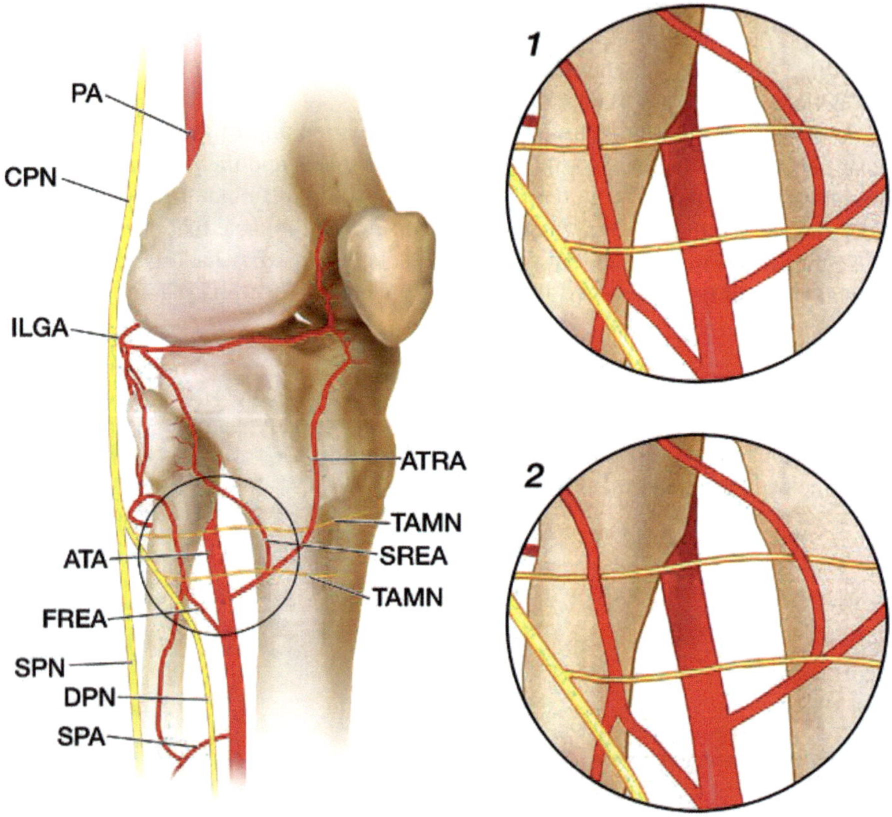

Fig. 2.5 Variations in the anatomical relationships between the motor nerves and the first and second recurrent epiphyseal vessels are demonstrated. *ATA* anterior tibial artery, *ATRA* anterior tibial recurrent artery, *CPN* common peroneal nerve, *DPN* distal peroneal nerve, *FREA* first recurrent epiphyseal artery, *ICGA* inferior lateral genicular artery, *PA* popliteal artery, *SPA* superficial peroneal artery, *SPN* superficial peroneal nerve, *SREA* second recurrent epiphyseal artery, *TAMN* tibialis anterior motor nerve. (Reprinted with permission from Mayo Foundation for Medical Education and Research. All rights reserved)

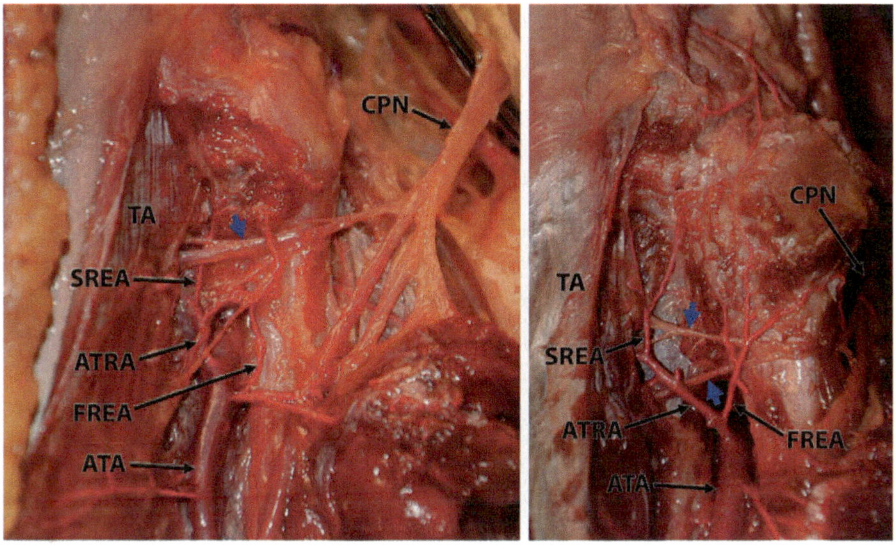

Fig. 2.6 Two examples illustrate the relation of the deep peroneal nerve branches to the tibialis anterior muscle in two specimens. One branch (*blue arrow*) courses deep to the first recurrent epiphyseal artery and superficial to the second recurrent epiphyseal artery (*left*). In the second specimen (*right*), two branches (*blue arrows*) travel deep beneath the first recurrent epiphyseal artery, the second recurrent epiphyseal artery, and the anterior tibial recurrent artery. *ATA* anterior tibial artery, *ATRA* anterior tibial recurrent artery, *FREA* first recurrent epiphyseal artery, *SREA* second recurrent epiphyseal artery, *CPN* common peroneal nerve, *TA* tibialis anterior muscle. (Copyright © 2018 by the American Society of Plastic Surgeons. Reprinted with permission from Morsy et al. [4]. All rights reserved)

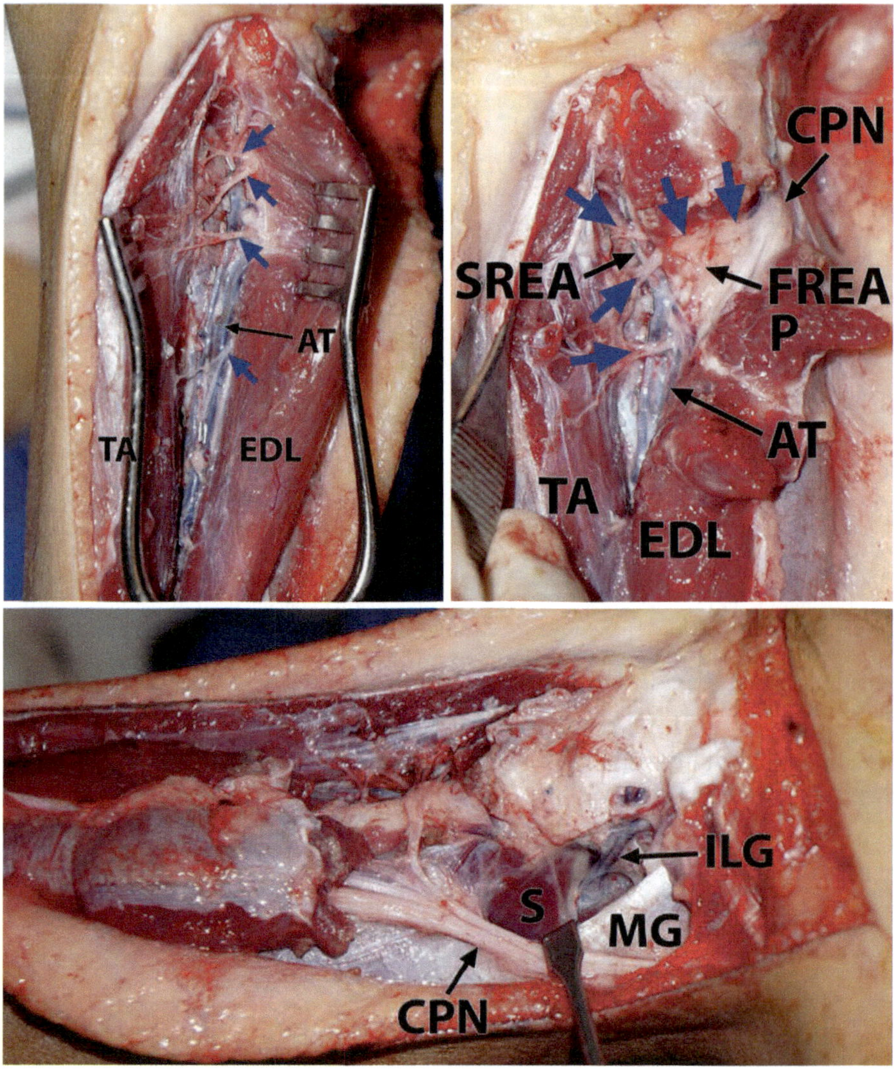

Fig. 2.7 Intraoperative photographs of the harvest of the proximal fibula for epiphyseal transfer. The upper left image shows the anterior tibial vessels located in the interval between the tibialis anterior and extensor digitorum longus muscles, crossed by motor nerves (*blue arrows*). The upper right image highlights the first and second recurrent epiphyseal arteries and their relationship to the motor nerves (*blue arrows*). The lower image displays the inferior lateral genicular vessels originating from the posterior aspect of the popliteal vessels. *AT* anterior tibial vessels, *FREA* first recurrent epiphyseal artery, *SREA* second recurrent epiphyseal artery, *ILG* inferior lateral genicular vessels, *CPN* common peroneal nerve, *TA* tibialis anterior muscle, *EDL* extensor digitorum longus, *P* peroneal muscle group, *S* soleus muscle, *MG* medial head of gastrocnemius.

Dissection Technique

The standard technique for harvesting the proximal fibular was described by Innocenti et al. [14] The patient was positioned supine and the hip and knee joints are flexed. We prefer the use of a sterile tourniquet for this procedure applied to the thigh for better exposure. A longitudinal skin incision is made centered over the anterolateral compartment in the lower leg. The incision is extended proximally, curving laterally over the fibular head and then more proximally following the biceps tendon (Fig. 2.8). The deep fascia of the anterolateral compartment distally is divided sharply longitudinally along the line of the incision at the interval between the tibialis anterior muscle and the extensor digitorum longus muscle. Blunt dissection is performed in between these muscles, separating them, and through this interval, the anterior tibial vessels and the deep peroneal nerve are exposed. Care is taken not to dissect along the lateral side of the vessels at this point in time, in order to preserve the periosteal branches to the shaft. Any motor branches coming from the deep peroneal nerve to the anterolateral compartment

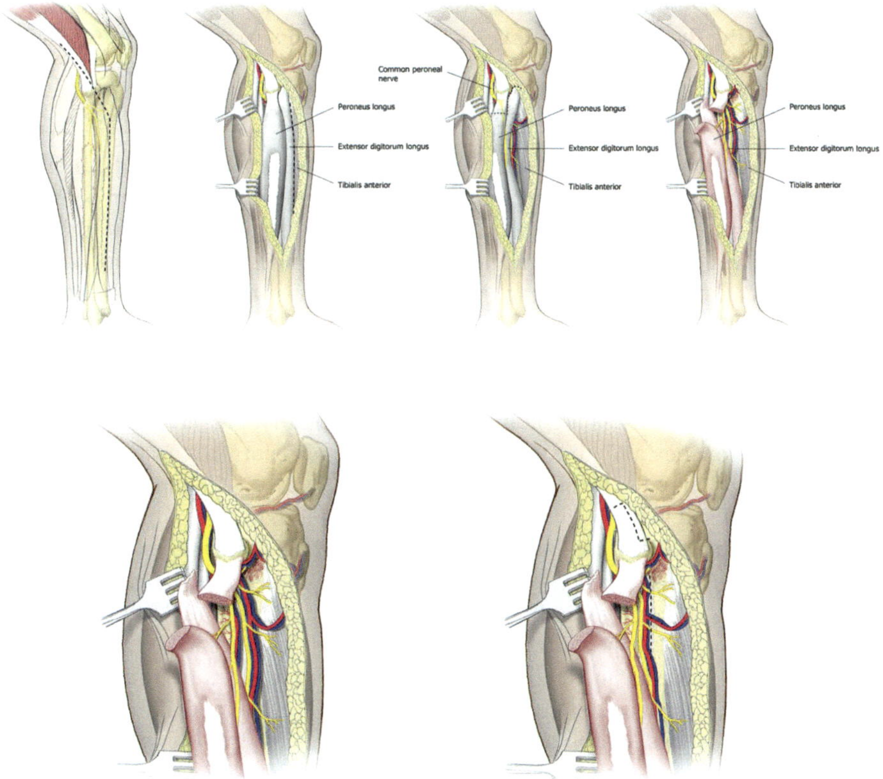

Fig. 2.8 Illustrations showing the surgical incision and detailed anatomy

muscles are meticulously dissected and preserved. The anterior tibial vessels and the deep peroneal nerve are dissected from distal to proximal towards the head of the fibula developing the interval further. At the level of the neck of the fibula, the extensor digitorum longus and the peroneus longus muscles are divided sharply, positioned superficial to the deep peroneal nerve and, more proximally, the common peroneal nerve. The cuff of muscle over the head of the fibula is preserved with the flap as it contains the recurrent epiphyseal vessels and there are smaller branches which are part of the anastomosis around the head of the fibula. Similar to the distal motor nerve branches, branches coming out from the deep peroneal nerve to the muscles need to be meticulously dissected and preserved. Some of the motor branches in the proximal and distal section may need to be divided for safely harvesting the pedicle. These will need to be repaired using microsurgical techniques. The extensor digitorum longus and peroneus longus muscles are dissected sharply distal to the nerve, exposing the fibula leaving a cuff of 1–2 mm thick of muscle over the fibula and the interosseous membrane to the desired length of the fibular shaft. This cuff of muscle serves to protect the periosteal branches from the anterior tibial vessels. The interosseous membrane is now divided sharply longitudinally medial to the anterior tibial vessels and kept attached to the fibula. This portion of the interosseous membrane will be harvested with the flap and care is taken not to dissect this from the vessels. The fibula is osteotomized at the desired length and an extra length of periosteum can be harvested distal to the osteotomy site to be used to overlap bone repair at the recipient site for better bone healing. The capsule of the proximal tibiofibular joint is now divided carefully. The lateral collateral ligament is divided off the fibular head as distal as possible and tagged. If a portion of the biceps tendon is required to be a part of the flap, the biceps tendon is divided longitudinally and the posterior half included in the anterior of the divided fibular head and tagged. If the inferior lateral macular vessels are visualized, they can be ligated and divided. A small bone clamp or a large Kelly forceps can be applied to the distal portion of the fibular shaft in order to allow for rotation of the fibula internally and externally to reset the remaining muscles as well as the peroneal vessels away from the flap. The anterior tibial vessels are now dissected proximally, preserving the recurrent epiphyseal branches and possibly the anterior tibial recurrent for as much length as possible and then the origin of the anterior tibial vessels from the tibioperoneal trunk are exposed. The distal part of the pedicle can be further dissected to gain more length and then it can be ligated and divided. The tourniquet is released to allow for reperfusion of the growth plate. We recommend reperfusion for about 20 minutes and bleeding can be observed from the muscle cuff surrounding the head. After adequate reperfusion, the anterior tibial vessels can be ligated at their origin and the harvest can be completed. Any motor branches from the deep peroneal nerve that had to be divided are now repaired. The lateral collateral ligaments as well as the biceps tendon are now sutured into the lateral tibia using a nonabsorbable transosseous stitch that can be reinforced with stitches into the surrounding periosteum. The wound is now closed in layers and the knee is immobilized for 4–6 weeks followed by full weight-bearing as tolerated.

Anastomosis

Anastomosis is performed in a reverse flow manner. The distal end of the anterior tibial artery is anastomosed, providing the arterial flow to the flap. The retrograde flow from the vein is usually adequate, provided that interconnections in between the two vena comitans are preserved during the harvest to bypass the valvular system [14, 20]. It is standard to perform the arterial anastomosis first and then a pause of about 10–20 min is customary to allow for the venous connection channels to open adequately to provide sufficient flow through the dominant vein. Usually, one vein will be sufficient to provide venous outflow from the flap.

Cases

Case 1

A 39-month-old male presented with a complete loss of the head and partial loss of the neck of the femur at the left hip consistent with a type IV late sequela of infantile septic arthritis of the hip. The hip was approached through an anterior Smith--Petersen approach. The head and the neck of the femur were reconstructed using a free vascularized epiphyseal transfer from the proximal fibula. The anastomosis was done between the lateral circumflex femoral vessels as the recipient site vessels to the anterior tibial vessels in a retrograde fashion. The 2-year and 5-year follow-up radiographs show progressive remodeling of the fibular head to fill the acetabular space. Clinically, the patient maintained a painless stable hip joint with an acceptable range of motion (Figs. 2.9 and 2.10).

Case 2

A 5-year-old female with loss of the lateral femoral condyle due to osteomyelitis of the distal femur 2 years prior to her presentation that led to destruction of the epiphysis and growth plate. She presented with a progressively worsening severe valgus deformity of the knee, which was exaggerated with weight-bearing. This was also accompanied by compensatory pelvic tilt and foot equinus. She underwent a vascularized fibular epiphyseal transfer from the contralateral lower extremity to reconstruct the lateral femoral condyle after correcting the valgus deformity, supplying a new growth plate and bony stability. The lateral collateral ligament was reconstructed by harvesting a portion of the biceps tendon. The anterior tibial vessels were anastomosed in a retrograde fashion to the superior lateral genicular vessels at the recipient site. At her 2-year follow-up, she has maintained the deformity correction and had a painless stable knee joint with a range of motion from 0° to 90°. The growth plate at the transferred fibular head was still open. The fibular head had remodeled to conform with the recipient site (Figs. 2.11, 2.12, 2.13, 2.14, 2.15, 2.16, and 2.17).

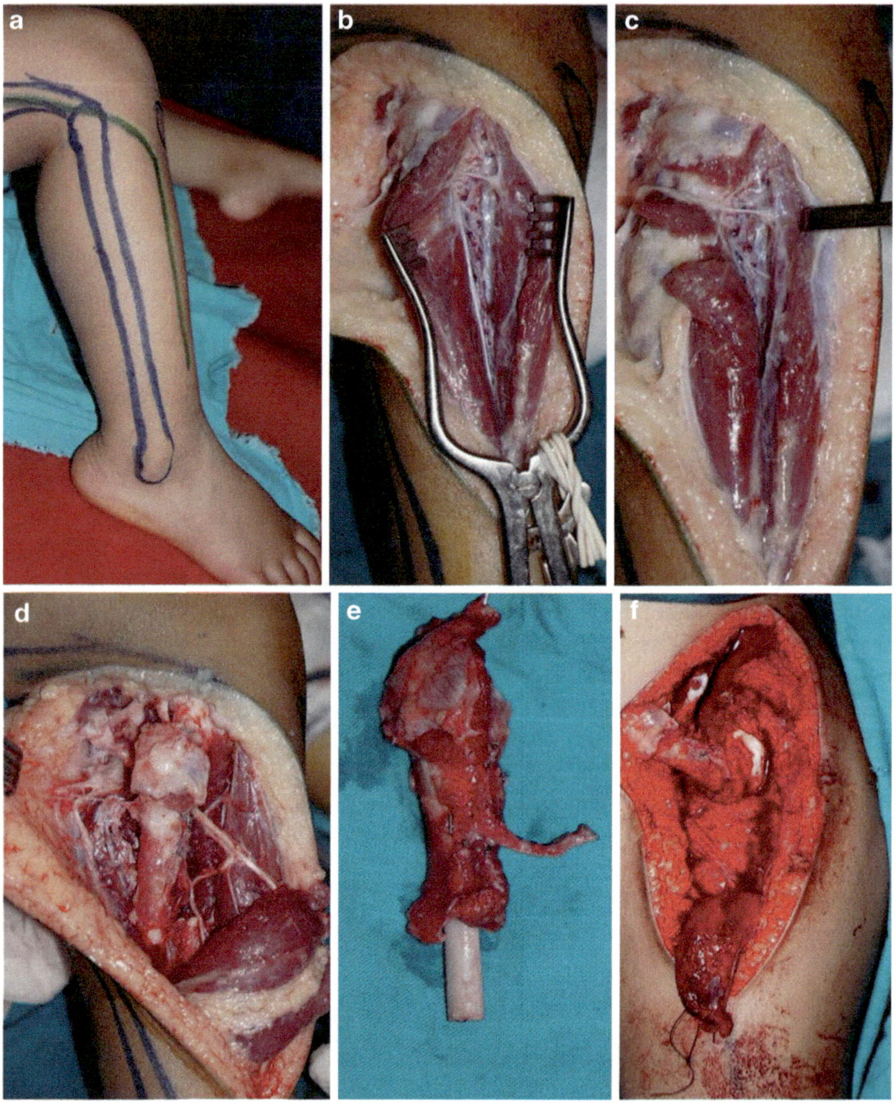

Fig. 2.9 Incision over the anterolateral leg, curving posteriorly over the fibular head and the biceps femoris tendon (**a**). The anterior tibial vessels are identified in the interval between the TA and the EDL muscles (**b**). Meticulous dissection of the peroneal nerve and its motor branches (**c**). Osteotomy of the fibula is performed after dissection of the muscle attachments off the bone (**d**). The proximal fibula after completion of the harvest (**e**). The proximal fibula doweled in the femur to replace the lost head and neck (**f**). EDL, extensor digitorum longus. (Copyright © 2024 Wolters Kluwer Health, Inc. Reprinted with permission from El-Gammal et al. [5]. All rights reserved)

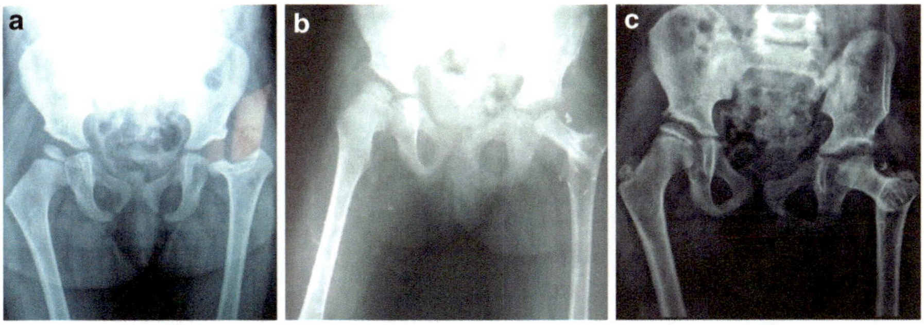

Fig. 2.10 A 39-month-old male with a type IVA late sequela of infantile septic arthritis of the left hip. Preoperative radiograph (**a**). Two-year follow-up radiograph (**b**). Five-year follow-up radiograph (**c**).

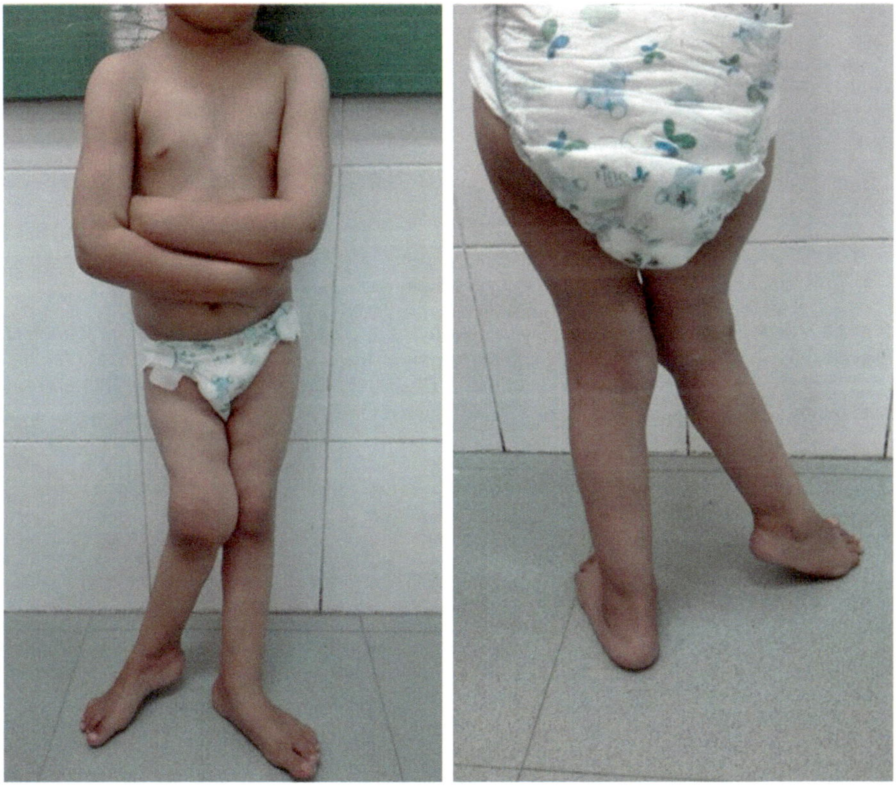

Fig. 2.11 Photographs show severe valgus deformity in the patient, as well as compensatory pelvic tilt and equinus deformity while standing.

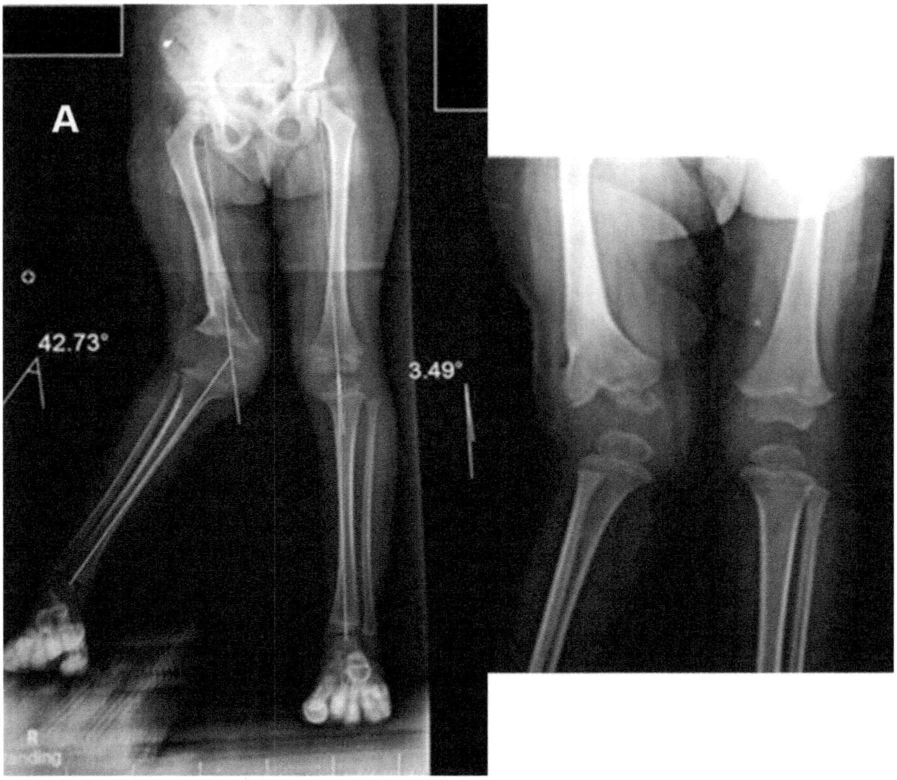

Fig. 2.12 X-Rays show a severe valgus deformity of 42.7° accompanied by a 6-cm leg length discrepancy (**a**). Imaging shows complete resorption of the ossific nucleus of the lateral femoral condyle (**b**). (Copyright © 2023 by The Journal of Bone and Joint Surgery, Incorporated. Reprinted with permission from El-Gammal et al. [1]. All rights reserved)

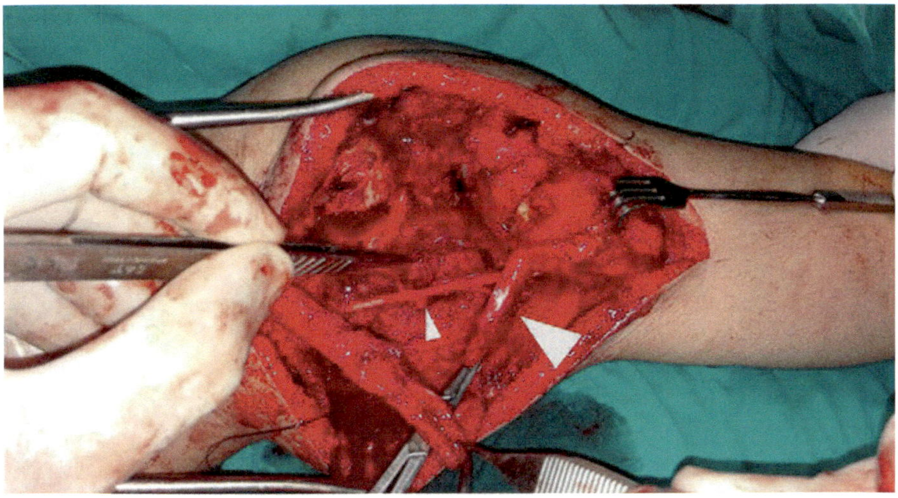

Fig. 2.13 Intraoperative photograph of the recipient's leg. The distal attachment of the lateral collateral ligament and biceps femoris tendon (*large arrow*). The common peroneal nerve (*small arrow*). Microforceps are pointing to the superior lateral genicular vessels.

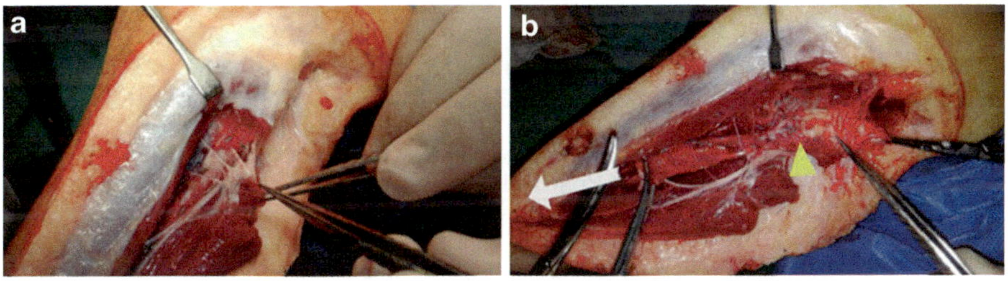

Fig. 2.14 All the nerve branches to the tibialis anterior muscle are identified. After osteotomizing the fibula, the anterior tibial vessels are clipped proximally, and the fibular epiphysis is withdrawn in a distal direction below the motor branches to the tibialis anterior muscles (**a**). The feeding vessels, typically originating from the anterior tibial vessels, are located on the posterior surface of the fibular head and neck (**b** *yellow arrow*).

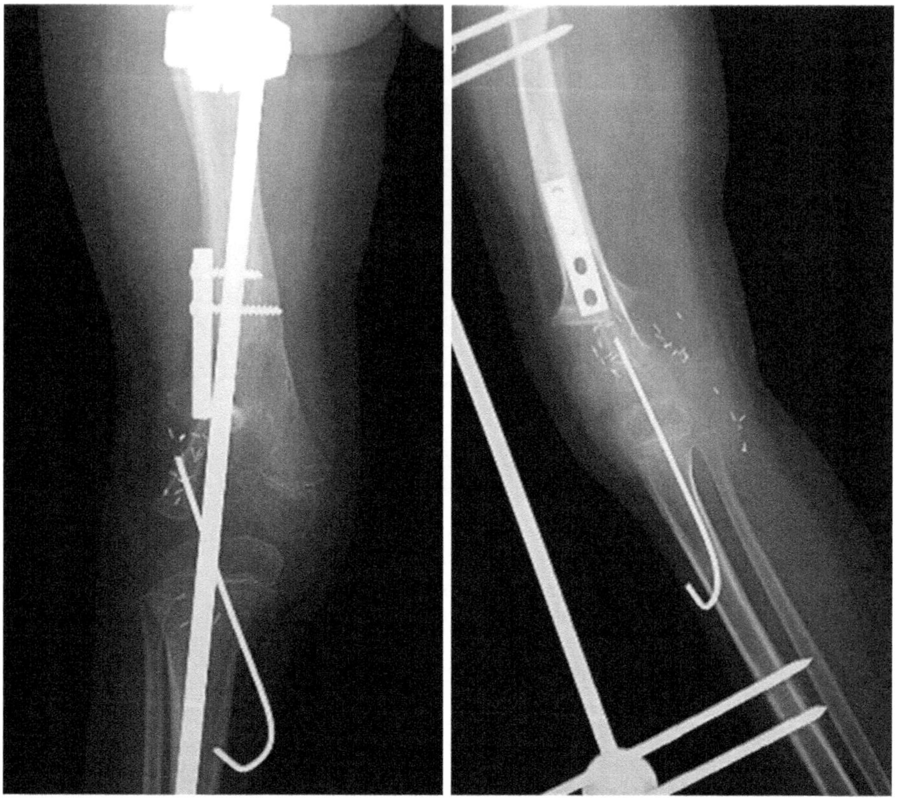

Fig. 2.15 X-Rays 6 weeks postoperatively show the union between the graft and the distal femur. (Copyright © 2023 by The Journal of Bone and Joint Surgery, Incorporated. Reprinted with permission from El-Gammal et al. [1]. All rights reserved)

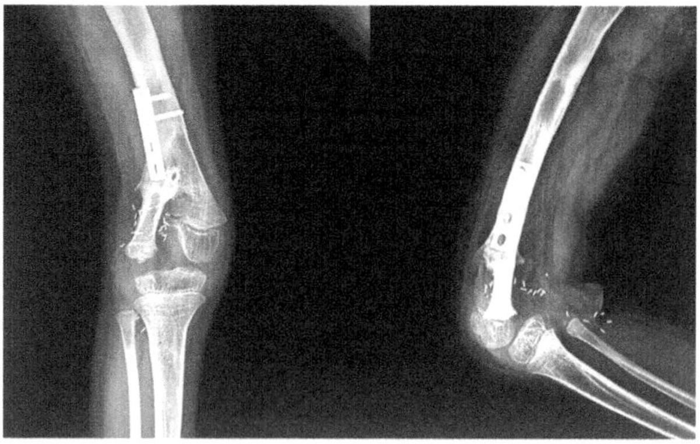

Fig. 2.16 X-Rays at the 2-year follow-up show successful bony consolidation of the transferred proximal fibula, with evidence of hypertrophy. The open epiphyseal plate and ossific nucleus of the transferred fibula are also demonstrated. (Copyright © 2023 by The Journal of Bone and Joint Surgery, Incorporated. Reprinted with permission from El-Gammal et al. [1]. All rights reserved)

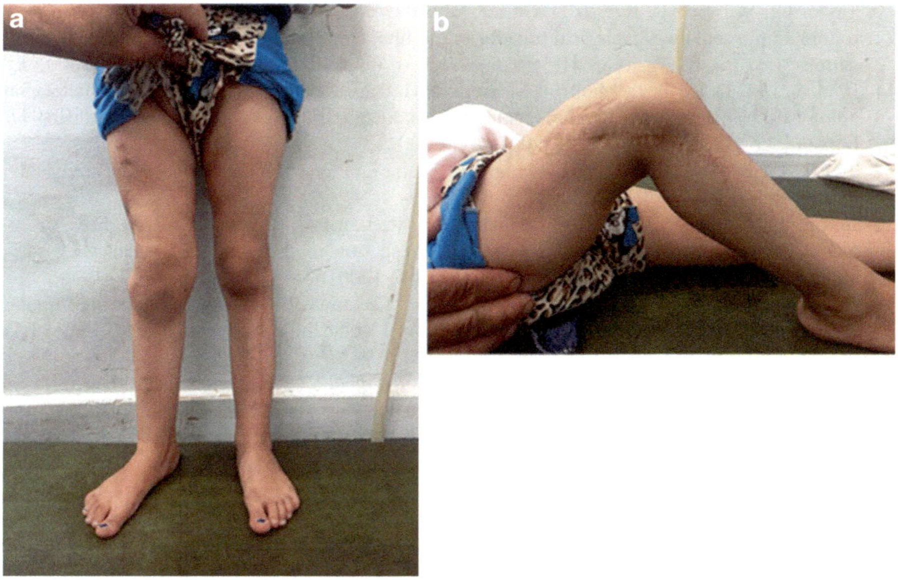

Fig. 2.17 Photographs at 2-year follow-up show the standing position (**a**) and active knee flexion (**b**). (Copyright © 2023 by The Journal of Bone and Joint Surgery, Incorporated. Reprinted with permission from El-Gammal et al. [1]. All rights reserved)

References

1. El-Gammal TA, Refai OA, Morsy M, Eisa AA. Reconstruction of a pediatric lateral femoral condyle after septic necrosis with a free vascularized fibular epiphysis: a case report. JBJS Case Connect. 2023;13(1):e22.00736. https://doi.org/10.2106/JBJS.CC.22.00736.
2. Innocenti M, Delcroix L, Balatri A. Vascularized growth plate transfer for distal radius reconstruction. Semin Plast Surg. 2008;22(3):186–94. https://doi.org/10.1055/s-2008-1081402.
3. Innocenti M, Delcroix L, Romano GF, Capanna R. Vascularized epiphyseal transplant. Orthop Clin North Am. 2007;38(1):95–101, vii. https://doi.org/10.1016/j.ocl.2006.10.003.
4. Morsy M, Sur YJ, Akdag O, Sabbagh MD, Suchyta MA, El-Gammal TA, et al. Vascularity of the proximal fibula and its implications in vascularized epiphyseal transfer: an anatomical and high-resolution computed tomographic angiography study. Plast Reconstr Surg. 2019;143(1):172e–83e. https://doi.org/10.1097/PRS.0000000000005127.
5. El-Gammal TA, El-Sayed Ali A, Kotb MM, Saleh WR, Ragheb YF, Refai OA, et al. Free vascularized proximal fibular epiphyseal transfer for hip reconstruction following septic necrosis in children. J Pediatr Orthop. 2024;44(5):308–15. https://doi.org/10.1097/BPO.0000000000002634.
6. Bowen CV, Singer S. Bernard O'Brien: the microsurgical transfer of immature bone. Microsurgery. 1994;15(10):733–7. https://doi.org/10.1002/micr.1920151013.
7. Boyer MI, Bray PW, Bowen CV. Epiphyseal plate transplantation: an historical review. Br J Plast Surg. 1994;47(8):563–9. https://doi.org/10.1016/0007-1226(94)90141-4.
8. Pho RW. Free vascularised fibular transplant for replacement of the lower radius. J Bone Joint Surg Br. 1979;61-B(3):362–5. https://doi.org/10.1302/0301-620X.61B3.479261.
9. Weiland AJ, Kleinert HE, Kutz JE, Daniel RK. Free vascularized bone grafts in surgery of the upper extremity. J Hand Surg Am. 1979;4(2):129–44. https://doi.org/10.1016/s0363-5023(79)80129-x.

10. Taylor GI, Wilson KR, Rees MD, Corlett RJ, Cole WG. The anterior tibial vessels and their role in epiphyseal and diaphyseal transfer of the fibula: experimental study and clinical applications. Br J Plast Surg. 1988;41(5):451–69. https://doi.org/10.1016/0007-1226(88)90001-x.
11. Innocenti M, Delcroix L, Manfrini M, Ceruso M, Capanna R. Vascularized proximal fibular epiphyseal transfer for distal radial reconstruction. J Bone Joint Surg Am. 2004;86(7):1504–11. https://doi.org/10.2106/00004623-200407000-00021.
12. Tsai TM, Ludwig L, Tonkin M. Vascularized fibular epiphyseal transfer. A clinical study. Clin Orthop Relat Res. 1986;210:228–34.
13. Innocenti M, Ceruso M, Manfrini M, Angeloni R, Lauri G, Capanna R, et al. Free vascularized growth-plate transfer after bone tumor resection in children. J Reconstr Microsurg. 1998;14(2):137–43. https://doi.org/10.1055/s-2007-1000157.
14. Innocenti M, Delcroix L, Manfrini M, Ceruso M, Capanna R. Vascularized proximal fibular epiphyseal transfer for distal radial reconstruction. J Bone Joint Surg Am. 2005;87 Suppl 1(Pt 2):237–46. https://doi.org/10.2106/JBJS.E.00295.
15. Innocenti M, Baldrighi C, Menichini G. Long term results of epiphyseal transplant in distal radius reconstruction in children. Handchir Mikrochir Plast Chir. 2015;47(2):83–9. https://doi.org/10.1055/s-0035-1547304.
16. Yang J, Qin B, Li P, Fu G, Xiang J, Gu L. Vascularized proximal fibular epiphyseal transfer for Bayne and Klug type III radial longitudinal deficiency in children. Plast Reconstr Surg. 2015;135(1):157e–66e. https://doi.org/10.1097/PRS.0000000000000836.
17. Restrepo J, Katz D, Gilbert A. Arterial vascularization of the proximal epiphysis and the diaphysis of the fibula. Int J Microsurg. 1980;2:49–54.
18. Bonnel F, Lesire M, Gomis R, Allieu Y, Rabischong P. Arterial vascularization of the fibula microsurgical transplant techniques – diaphysis – superior epiphysis. Anat Clin. 1981;3(1):13–22.
19. Mozaffarian K, Lascombes P, Dautel G. Vascular basis of free transfer of proximal epiphysis and diaphysis of fibula: an anatomical study. Arch Orthop Trauma Surg. 2009;129(2):183–7. https://doi.org/10.1007/s00402-008-0600-3.
20. del Pinal F, Taylor GI. The deep venous system and reverse flow flaps. Br J Plast Surg. 1993;46(8):652–64. https://doi.org/10.1016/0007-1226(93)90195-h.

Chapter 3
Bone and Cartilage Flaps from the Distal Femur

Ledibabari Mildred Ngaage and James Higgins

Introduction

The development of the common vascularized bone flaps in reconstructive surgery has historically occurred via two pathways. The first is when a full-thickness segment of donor tubular bone is harvested to reconstruct a similar tubular defect. This is made possible by the structural integrity that adjacent skeletal components afford the donor extremity (i.e., fibular flap, free toe flaps). The second pathway occurs when partial thickness segments of bone are harvested as chimeric components of common skin or muscle flaps due to the observed soft tissue attachments between the bone segment and the soft tissue flap (i.e., radius, scapula, distal humerus, and rib).

The evolution of the distal femur as a source of vascularized bone occurred via a novel pathway. Unlike the fibula harvest site, the femur cannot provide a source of full-thickness tubular bone due to its singular role in the structural integrity of the extremity. Unlike the scapular bone flap or radius bone flap, distal femur flaps did not evolve from the use of an adjacent soft tissue flap. The initial application of the unicortical flap from the medial side of the femur was in the form of a corticoperiosteal flap based on the observed dense filigree of periosteal vessels in the region associated with a lengthy axial pedicle. The initial descriptions of the pedicled [1] and free [2] unicortical MFC flaps were followed by numerous reports of clinical applications. Studies followed that described the vascular anatomy [3–6], chimeric applications [5, 7–9] and donor site considerations [10–13].

L. M. Ngaage
Department of Plastic and Reconstructive Surgery, Johns Hopkins School of Medicine, Baltimore, MD, USA

J. Higgins (✉)
Curtis National Hand Center, Medstar Union Memorial Hospital, Baltimore, MD, USA
e-mail: higgins@curtishand.com

J. P. Agarwal, D. W. Mathes (eds.), *Bone Flaps in Reconstructive Surgery*,
https://doi.org/10.1007/978-3-032-12540-8_3

The examination of the periosteal perfusion of this region led to the creation of other useful osseous flaps. The less commonly used LFC is harvested from the lateral face of the femur based on the superolateral geniculate artery system. The pedicle is shorter but provides generous caliber for microsurgical anastomoses. Like the MFC flap, the LFC flap provides options for the inclusion of skin and tendon segment and does not require the sacrifice of a major vessel to the distal extremity [14–16].

The periosteal vessels on both the medial and lateral side of the distal femur demonstrate branches that course to the proximal-most segment of convex cartilage of the medial trochlea and lateral trochlea, respectively. These cartilage segments of the femoral articular surface are areas that encounter very low contact pressures when articulating with the patella [17] and do not articulate with the tibia. This permits harvest of small vascularized osteochondral flaps for reconstruction of articular defects elsewhere in the human skeleton. The osteochondral MFT and LFT flaps are used most commonly for the treatment of extremely small fragmented scaphoid proximal pole nonunions [18, 19], or in advanced Kienbock's disease demonstrating significant fragmentation and collapse [20–24]. The anatomy of both flaps is consistent, and harvest can be performed with the patient in the supine position, permitting a two-surgeon approach.

Indications

Corticocancellous MFC and LFC Flaps

The MFC flap is commonly used for long bone nonunions throughout the skeleton. It can be harvested as a *corticocancellous* flap for small intercalary defects with acceptable donor site morbidity [10]. It does not provide structural bone as the unicortical surface harvested is thin and pliable. As a result, the applications are limited to defects where hardware can provide adequate structural support during the entire period of healing. The bone quality is ideal for rapid healing of small recalcitrant nonunions as it has a dense cancellous component and a rich vascular network on the overlying periosteum.

The MFC is also commonly harvested as a thin *corticoperiosteal* flap that may be used in cases of atrophic nonunion where there is minimal intercalary defect. The thin nature of the cortical face of the medial condyle permits bending of the flap and contouring over the surfaces of the nonunion site [7]. The length of the descending geniculate pedicle and the ease of harvest of a chimeric skin component makes the MFC corticocancellous flap more desirable than the LFC flap for long bone or tubular bone reconstruction [25].

There are many bone grafting and pedicle flap techniques described for the treatment of scaphoid nonunions. The MFC and LFC have demonstrated particular utility in cases that have failed previous surgical attempts at correction [26, 27]. In these cases, a small corticocancellous segment is placed at the nonunion site via a volar wrist approach. The reconstruction is fixed with either screw or Kirschner wire fixation driven retrograde, starting in the distal pole, passing through the intercalary flap, and terminating in the proximal pole. The proximity of the radial artery enables the use of a short vascular pedicle, making both MFC and LFC useful options. The MFC or LFC is selected if the proximal pole fragment is deemed adequate to preserve. If the proximal pole is not salvageable due to excessive fragmentation or small size, the use of the MFC or LFC is contraindicated, and consideration is given to osteochondral flap reconstruction [28–30].

Osteochondral MFT and LFT Flaps

MFT and LFT flaps provide vascularized osteochondral convex surfaces for the reconstruction of morphologically similar articular surfaces [31, 32]. While both are convex, their morphology is different, making each better suited to particular defects.

The proximal pole segment of recalcitrant scaphoid nonunions is deemed nonsalvageable if it is highly fragmented from previous instrumentation, or too small to provide purchase for fixation. In this setting, patients are considered potential candidates for osteochondral reconstruction with either the MFT or LFT flap [30, 33, 34]. The second most common application of the MFT flap is for the reconstruction of the proximal lunate in cases of collapse and fragmentation without arthritic changes in the capitate or radius surfaces [22, 23, 35].

Less common indications for osteochondral flap reconstruction include proximal capitate avascular necrosis (without arthritic changes on the other surfaces of the midcarpal joint) and avascular necrosis of the talus. In these settings, the defects are better suited for a segment of bone that has a more acute angle between the cartilage-bearing surface and the cortical surface. The LFT morphology best fits these requirements and provides an excellent restoration of the proximal capitate and proximal-medial talus [8, 36].

In addition to the morphological considerations, the senior author also maintains additional requirements for candidacy for osteochondral harvest from the distal femur. These include skeletal maturity, patient age <40 years, and BMI <35.

Anatomy and Dissection

Medial Femoral Condyle (MFC) Flap

The medial femoral condyle is perfused most commonly by osteoarticular periosteal branches of the descending geniculate artery, which arises from the superficial femoral artery in the proximal aspect of the adductor canal (Fig. 3.1). The

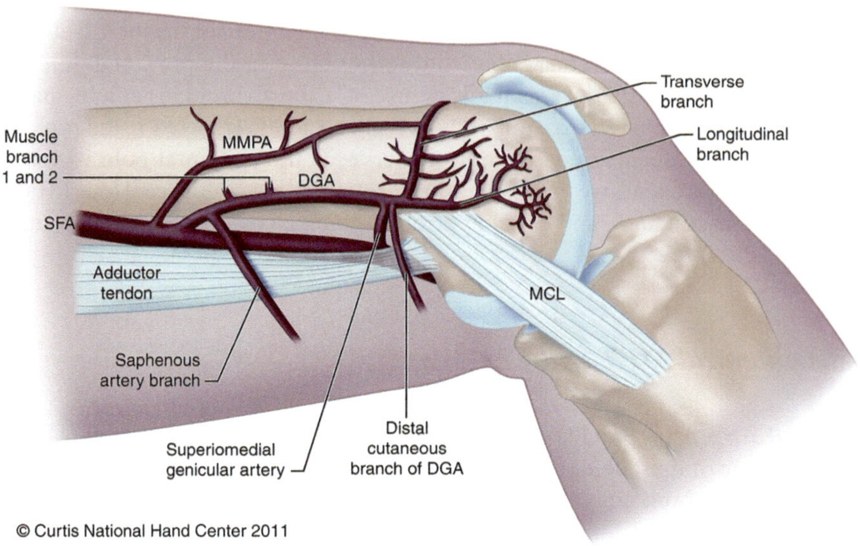

Fig. 3.1 Diagram of the arterial anatomy of the medial femur. The MFC flap is based on the longitudinal branch of the DGA, whereas the MFT flap is based on the transverse branch of the DGA. A skin component may be harvested with the MFC using the saphenous artery branch or distal cutaneous branch of the DGA. In 11% of cases the DGA may be absent and the periosteal system may be harvested based on the superomedial geniculate artery arising from the popliteal fossa. *DGA* descending geniculate artery, *MCL* medial collateral ligament, *MMPA* medial metaphyseal periosteal artery, *SFA* superficial femoral artery

descending geniculate artery may be absent in 11% of cases [4]. In this instance, these osteoarticular branches covering the periosteum of the medial femoral condyle are fed by the superomedial geniculate artery arising from the popliteal artery [7]. Familiarity with this vascular system enables the surgeon to first identify the periosteal branches and then follow them proximally to the appropriate source vessel.

The medial femoral condyle flap is often harvested with a skin component. The skin may be harvested using the saphenous artery branch of the descending geniculate artery or the distal cutaneous branches. This enables the surgeon to harvest a longitudinal ellipse of skin over the medial aspect of the thigh. This region may provide generous amounts of skin while still readily permitting primary closure [5, 9].

The descending geniculate artery has a length of 9.1–9.9 cm from its origin to the periosteal branches and at its origin has a diameter of 2.1 mm. The average diameter of the associated veins is 1.48–1.63 mm. If the flap is harvested utilizing the superomedial geniculate artery, the surgeon will encounter a vessel whose average length is 4.1 cm with an average diameter of 1.7 mm [5, 6].

Operative Technique

The patient is placed supine with the knee flexed and hip externally rotated in a frog leg position. The leg is prepped and draped up to the groin crease. A sterile tourniquet is utilized at the proximal thigh level. The skin incision used depends on the requirements of the case. If no skin is needed, a simple straight line is made between the palpable prominence of the medial condyle and the adductor canal. Alternatively, if a skin component is needed, a curvilinear incision is made on the medial thigh from the adductor hiatus to the midpoint between the medial border of the patella and the medial femoral condyle (Fig. 3.2). The muscular fascia is incised and the vastus medialis is retracted anteriorly, exposing the medial face of the femur and permitting a view of the periosteal vessels. The DGA may be identified originating from the SFA at the adductor hiatus, coursing along the adductor tendon, and investing into periosteum of the distal femur. The DGA divides into a longitudinal periosteal branch that drapes over the prominent apex of the medial condyle. The transverse branch courses anteriorly toward the medial trochlea. When harvesting the corticocancellous MFC, the transverse branch is ligated and the longitudinal branch of the DGA is preserved. Skin branches from the DGA (which include the saphenous artery) provide options for skin paddle harvest. In cases where the DGA is absent, the periosteal vessels can be followed proximally to the superomedial geniculate artery (SMGA) arising from the popliteal fossa [37, 38].

If a skin paddle component is desired, the surgeon now selects the desired branch of the vascular pedicle to support the skin component. The most employed branch is the saphenous artery branch, although reliable skin harvest may be performed using the distal cutaneous perforator of the DGA system. Prior to harvesting the bone component, the surgeon should complete the elevation of the skin paddle by elevating a longitudinal ellipse of skin using the initial skin incision as the anterior border of the skin flap segment. Once the skin paddle is elevated solely on the

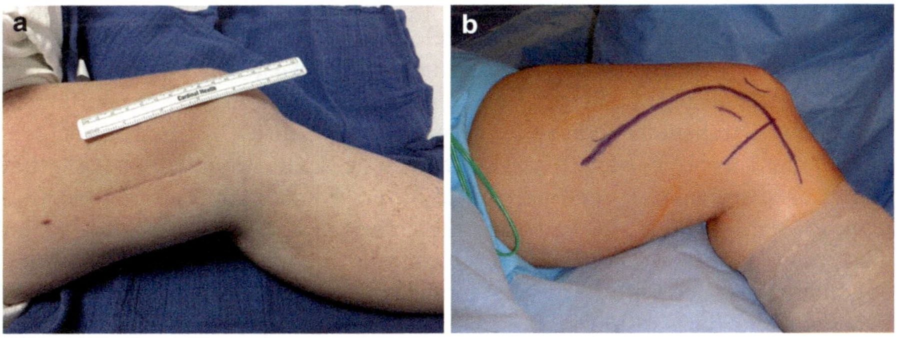

Fig. 3.2 (**a**) Incision for the medial femoral condyle (MFC) flap if no skin component is planned. (**b**) If a skin component is required, a curvilinear incision is made on the medial thigh from the adductor hiatus to the midpoint between the medial border of the patella and the medial condyle

cutaneous vessel, it is useful to deflate the tourniquet. This enables the surgeon to confirm viability of the skin paddle harvest prior to proceeding with the bone harvest. The bone harvest is simplified by proximal ligation and mobilization of the vascular pedicle, making subsequent confirmation of the skin paddle perfusion impossible.

After affirming skin vitality, the leg is exsanguinated again, and the tourniquet is inflated. The DGA or SMGA vascular pedicle is ligated proximally and reflected distally. The dimensions of the desired corticocancellous flap are measured and the thin cortical bone is scored using a sagittal saw. Osteotomes are used to complete elevation of the bone segment. In cases where intercalary bone is needed, the underlying cancellous bone is carefully included in the harvest. Alternatively, if a thin corticoperiosteal flap is needed, the layer may be elevated using a curved osteotome passed immediately beneath the cortex. After the flap is placed on the back table, gel foam is applied to the cancellous surface of the donor site and the skin closed in layers over a closed suction drain. The donor site does not require postoperative splinting or immobilization.

Medial Femoral Trochlea (MFT) Flap

The MFT harvest is similar to the MFC harvest with a few notable differences. When harvesting the MFT for carpal reconstruction, a skin paddle is usually not utilized. The incision is a 7.5-cm straight line starting over the palpable medial trochlea and coursing proximally and posteriorly in the direction of the adductor canal. The dissection then continues in a similar fashion as the MFC to expose the same vascular pedicle [30] (Fig. 3.3).

In order to harvest the MFT, the joint capsule is opened and the proximal and medial most segment of convex cartilage is visualized. The transverse branch of the DGA is invested into the periosteum surrounding this segment and will serve as the periosteal pedicle. Thus, the longitudinal branch is ligated, and the transverse branch is included in harvest. The DGA (or SMGA if the DGA is absent) pedicle is ligated proximally. As the pedicle is reflected distally, the transverse branch is elevated subperiosteally to the trochlea. Three bone cuts are needed to harvest the osteochondral component. A sagittal saw is used to make the coronal and transverse bone cuts. The final sagittal plane cut is made with a curved osteotome inserted with meticulous care under the retracted patella. The flap is removed, and the cancellous surface of the donor site is treated with fibrin glue to minimize surface bleeding. The joint is irrigated, and the capsule is closed. A drain is placed in the subcutaneous plane and the skin is closed in layers. The donor site does not require postoperative splinting or immobilization. This procedure has most commonly been performed for reconstruction of the recalcitrant scaphoid proximal pole nonunion and reconstruction of the proximal lunate in cases of advanced Kienbock's disease [34, 39–41] (Fig. 3.4).

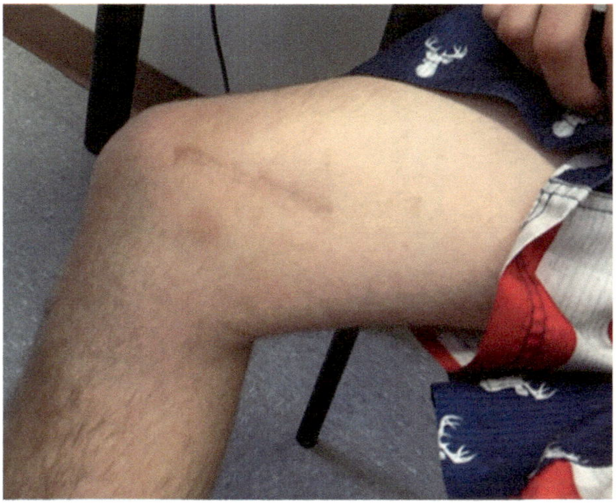

Fig. 3.3 Trajectory and length of skin incision used to harvest an MFT flap for articular reconstruction

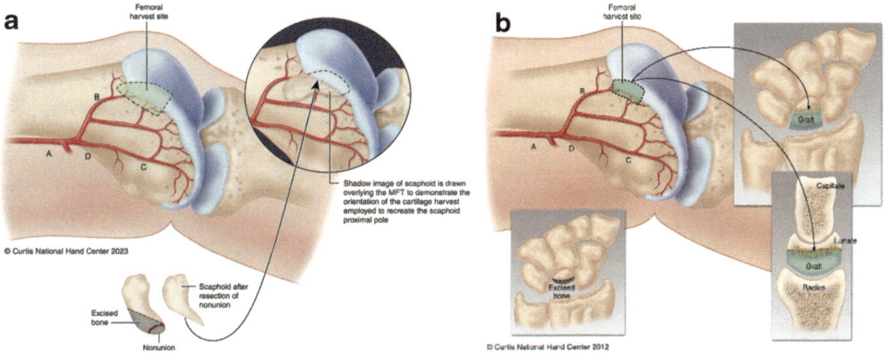

Fig. 3.4 Diagrammatic representation of the MFT procedure utilized for reconstruction of the proximal scaphoid (left) and proximal lunate (right). *A* descending geniculate artery; *B* transverse branch; *C* longitudinal branch; *D* superomedial geniculate artery

Lateral Femoral Condyle (LFC) and Lateral Femoral Trochlea (LFT) Flaps

The LFC and LFT flaps are based on the superolateral geniculate artery (SLGA) which originates from the popliteal artery at approximately 5 cm proximal to the knee joint (Fig. 3.5). It has a pedicle length of 5 cm and a diameter of 1.8 mm [14, 15]. The SLGA gives off perforators in a triangular area bordered by the LFC, vastus lateralis, and short head of the biceps femoris [14]. The inferior branch can be sacrificed to increase pedicle length. The vascularized iliotibial band can be harvested concurrently to provide composite transfer of tendon and bone [15]. Inclusion of a skin paddle with the LFC is possible if the periosteal system provides a favorable cutaneous perforator. This is unpredictable due to the variable cutaneous vascular anatomy.

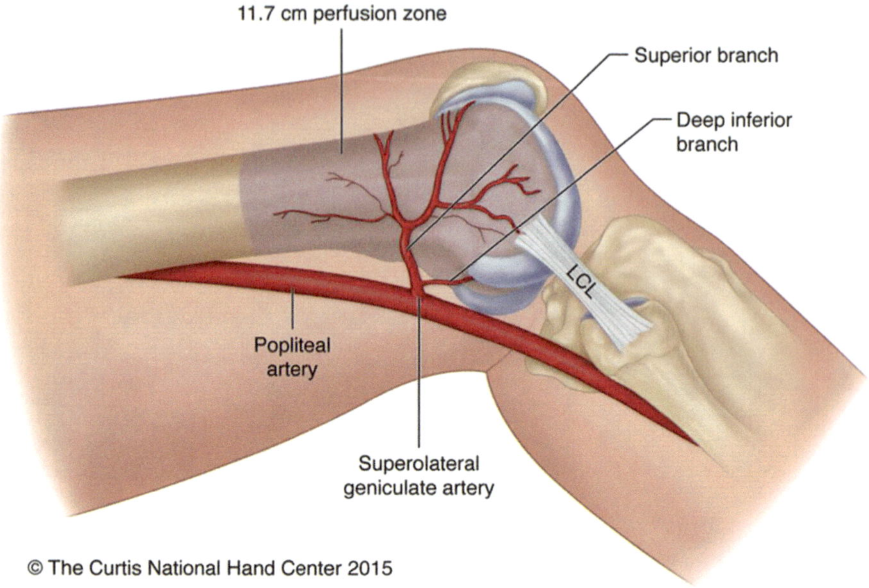

Fig. 3.5 Vascular anatomy of the periosteal vessels supplying the lateral distal femur. In this location the superolateral geniculate artery is the consistent vascular pedicle

Operative Technique

The patient is placed supine with the knee flexed and hip internally rotated with padding placed under the ipsilateral hip. The leg is prepped and draped up to the groin crease. A sterile tourniquet is utilized at the proximal thigh level. A longitudinal incision is made from the lateral femoral trochlea and the popliteal fossa. A window is made in the sheetlike fascia over the vastus lateralis, preserving the more posterior and thicker iliotibial band (Fig. 3.6). The vastus lateralis muscle is identified and retracted anteriorly, exposing the lateral face of the femoral condyle and the overlying periosteal vessels. The periosteal vessels converge into the single SLGA posteriorly. This source vessel is identified and dissected proximally into the

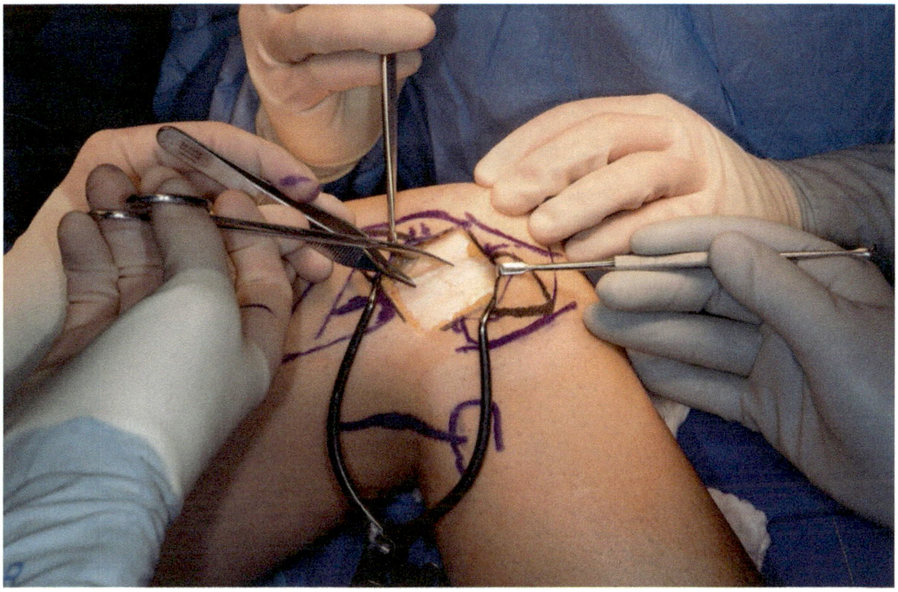

Fig. 3.6 After opening the skin via a straight incision from the lateral trochlea to the popliteal fossa, a thick sheet of fascia overlying the vastus lateralis is incised to expose the lateral trochlea. The thickened posterior iliotibial band is preserved

popliteal fossa. When adequate length is obtained, it is ligated and reflected anteriorly to the region of bone to be harvested [14, 24]. In a similar fashion to the MFC, the corticocancellous flap is elevated using a sagittal saw and osteotomes. If an osteochondral LFT flap is needed, the joint capsule is opened, and the same vascular pedicle is followed to the periosteum and perichondrium of the LFT. The LFT is harvested similarly to the MFT [16]. The joint capsule is then closed, a closed suction drain is placed in the subcutaneous plane, and the skin is closed. Patients are permitted to ambulate immediately after surgery. The osteochondral LFT procedure has been used for scaphoid nonunion surgery in a similar manner to the MFT. It has also been demonstrated to be a useful tool in the reconstruction of the proximal capitate (Fig. 3.7).

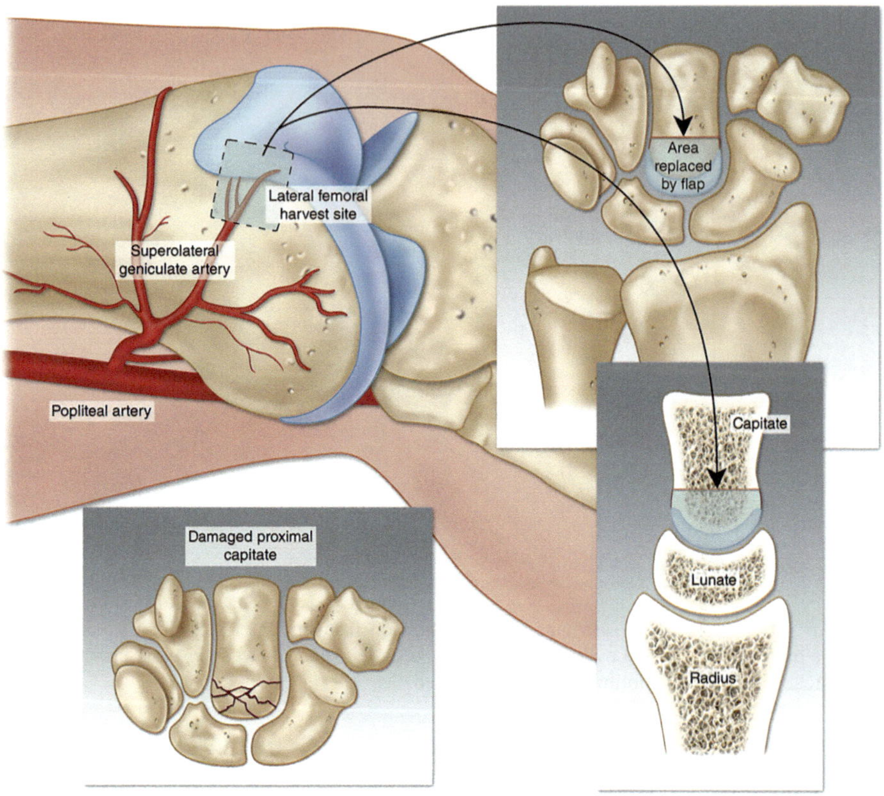

Fig. 3.7 Diagram of lateral femoral trochlea (LFT) reconstruction of the proximal capitate. The damaged proximal capitate is resected and the LFT is used to reconstruct the convex proximal capitate surface using the superolateral geniculate artery as the vascular pedicle

Case Example 1

A 65-year-old right-hand-dominant woman presented with a nonunion of her right radius metaphysis 9 months after undergoing unsuccessful management of a fracture at an outside hospital via a dorsal approach. X-rays demonstrated a healed ulnar fracture and index metacarpal fracture. Her radius nonunion demonstrated hardware failure, apex-dorsal angulation, and ulnar positive variance (Fig. 3.8). The patient underwent a revision fixation via a volar approach with locking plate fixation. A corticocancellous MFC flap was placed in the intercalary defect with the cortex oriented radially (Fig. 3.9a–c). The skin paddle emerged volarly along the FCR incision, and the anastomosis was performed end-to-side into the radial artery. After X-rays showed bony healing, the skin paddle was electively removed for contour restoration. By 14 months post-surgery, X-rays demonstrated healing and restoration of alignment with ulnar negative variance (Fig. 3.10).

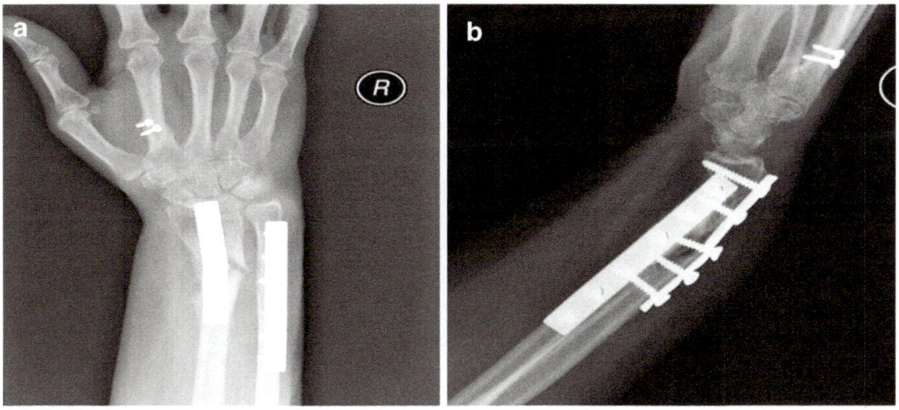

Fig. 3.8 Preoperative anteroposterior (**a**) and lateral (**b**) X-ray demonstrating distal radius metaphyseal nonunion, a healed ulnar fracture, and healed index metacarpal fracture. The radius nonunion demonstrates hardware failure, apex-dorsal angulation, and ulnar positive variance

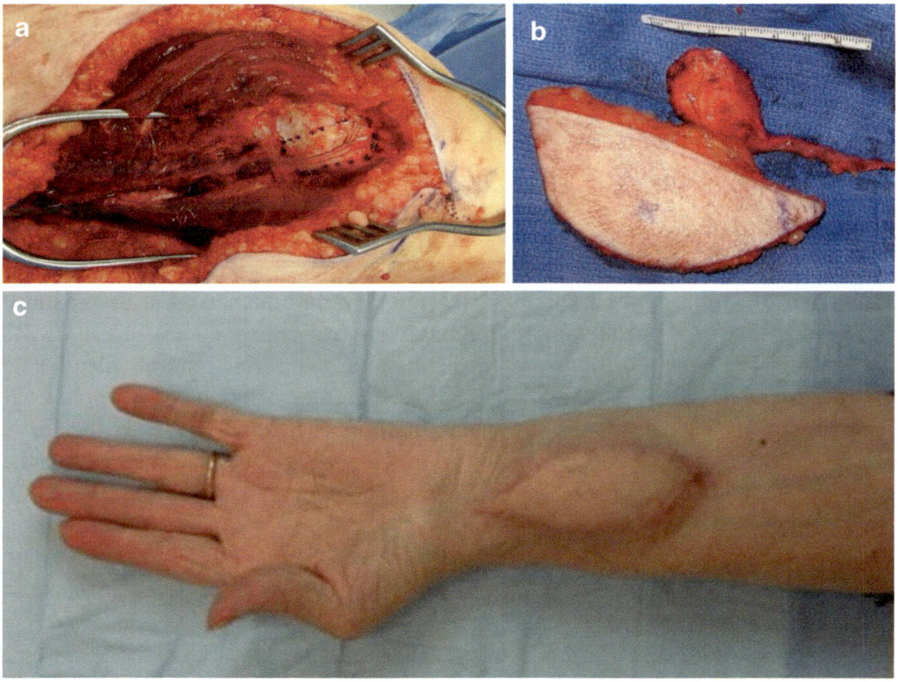

Fig. 3.9 (**a**) The vascular pedicle and bone segment are marked after the medial face of the femur was exposed by elevation of the vastus medialis muscle. (**b**) A corticocancellous MFC flap was harvested with a skin paddle. (**c**) The skin paddle inset along the volar approach incision

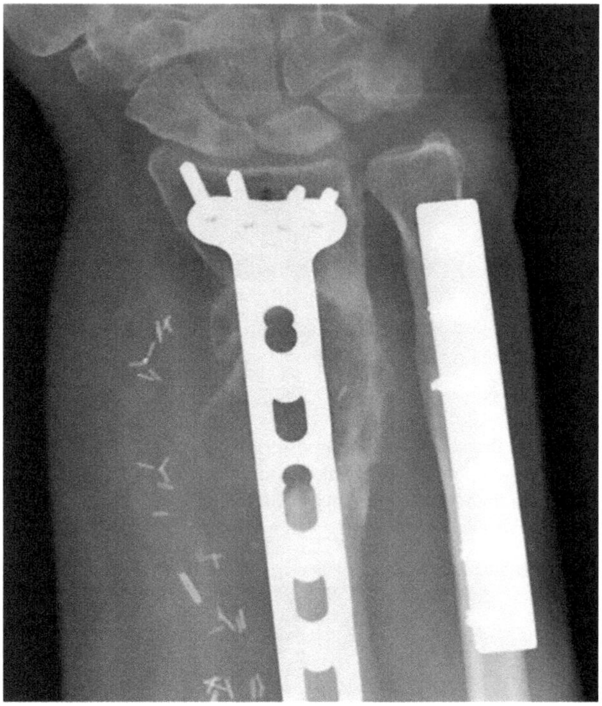

Fig. 3.10 Postoperative X-rays at 14 months demonstrate healing and restoration of alignment and ulnar negative variance

Case Example 2

A 24-year-old right-hand-dominant male automechanic presented with a painful recalcitrant proximal pole scaphoid nonunion. He had been treated years ago with nonvascularized bone grafting from his distal radius and screw fixation via a dorsal approach. The patient's X-ray demonstrated an extremely small proximal pole fragment and CT scan displayed fragmentation of the remaining proximal pole (Fig. 3.11). He was treated with resection of the proximal pole to the level of the scaphoid waist while preserving the concave acetabulum of the scaphoid (Fig. 3.12a, b). The proximal pole was replaced with a vascularized MFT flap with screw fixation (Fig. 3.13). Long-term X-rays demonstrate successful union, good preservation of carpal alignment, and no development of arthritic changes in the radioscaphoid articulation (Fig. 3.14b).

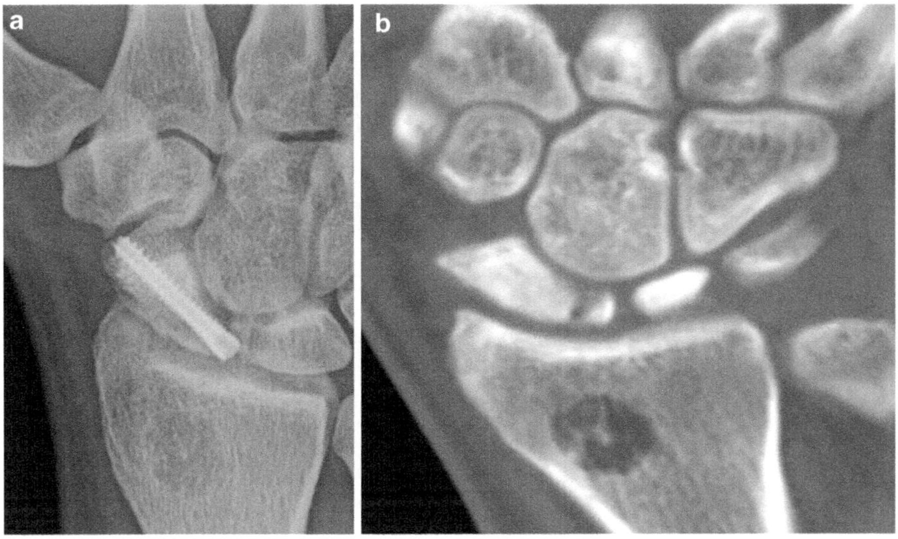

Fig. 3.11 (**a**) Preoperative X-ray demonstrating recalcitrant nonunion of the scaphoid proximal pole. The nonunion was previously treated with nonvascularized bone grafting from the distal radius and screw fixation. (**b**) Preoperative CT scan coronal images demonstrating the extremely small remaining proximal pole fragment which was deemed non-salvageable by conventional methods

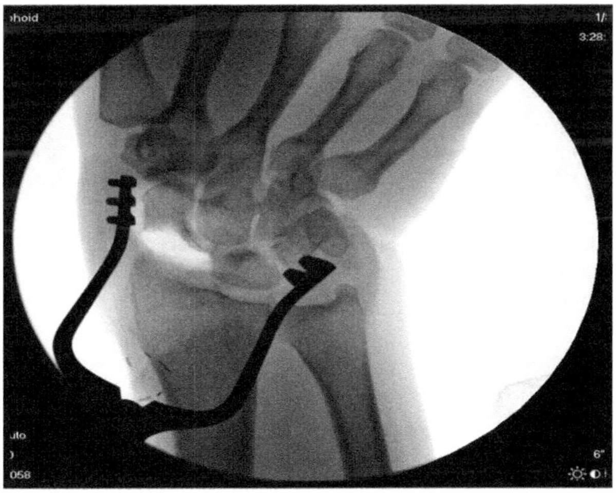

Fig. 3.12 Intraoperative fluoroscopy demonstrating the proximal pole was resected to the level of the scaphoid waist. The concave acetabulum of the scaphoid articulating with the capitate is preserved

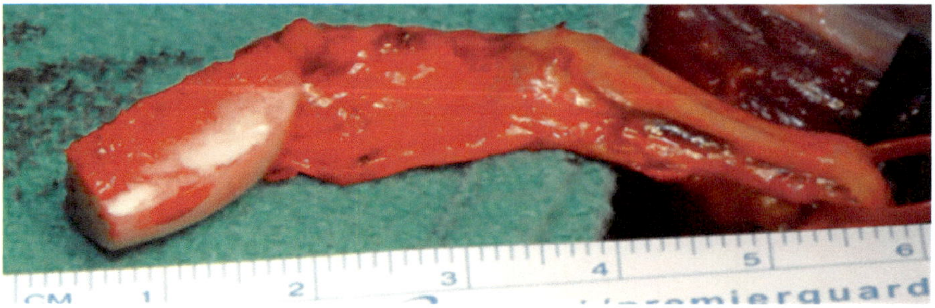

Fig. 3.13 Appearance of the harvested MFT osteochondral flap and pedicle. Note the thick layer of convex cartilage that is used to recreate the greater curvature of the proximal scaphoid

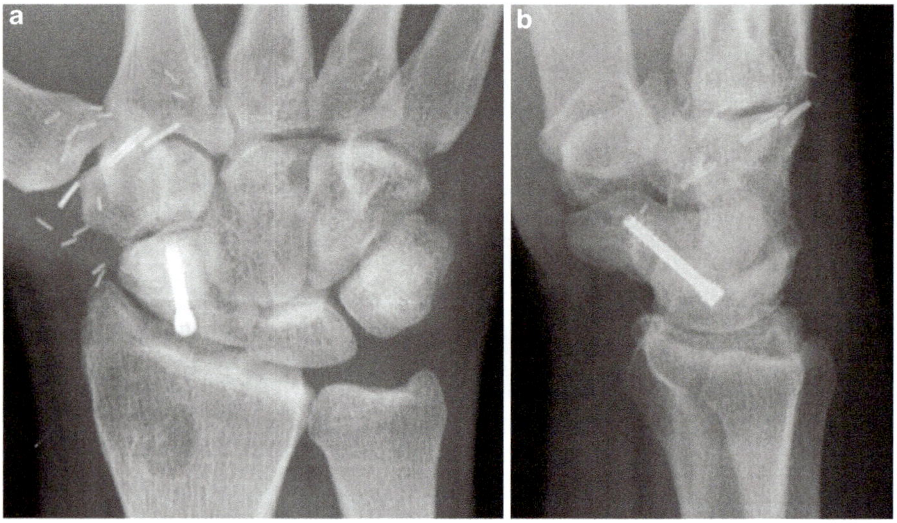

Fig. 3.14 Postoperative anteroposterior (**a**) and lateral (**b**) radiographs demonstrate successful union and good preservation of carpal alignment. No arthritic changes in the radioscaphoid articulation are present

Summary

The vascular anatomy of the periosteum of the distal femur provides the opportunity to harvest unicortical, corticocancellous, and corticoperiosteal bone flaps as well as small convex osteochondral flaps based on noncritical regional periosteal vascular pedicles. The anatomy, versatility, and applications of these flaps have been an area of exploration and innovation in reconstructive plastic surgery over the past 30 years. Familiarity with the vascular anatomy, harvest technique, chimeric options, and osteology of this region provides opportunities for intra-articular and extra-articular applications throughout the human skeleton.

References

1. Masquelet AC, Nordin JY, Guinot A. Vascularized transfer of the adductor magnus tendon and its osseous insertion: a preliminary report. J Reconstr Microsurg. 1985;1(3):169–76. https://doi.org/10.1055/s-2007-1007071.
2. Sakai K, Doi K, Kawai S. Free vascularized thin corticoperiosteal graft. Plast Reconstr Surg. 1991;87(2):290–8. https://doi.org/10.1097/00006534-199102000-00011.
3. Hugon S, Koninckx A, Barbier O. Vascularized osteochondral graft from the medial femoral trochlea: anatomical study and clinical perspectives. Surg Radiol Anat. 2010;32(9):817–25.
4. Yamamoto H, Jones DB Jr, Moran SL, Bishop AT, Shin AY. The arterial anatomy of the medial femoral condyle and its clinical implications. J Hand Surg Eur. 2010;35(7):569–74. https://doi.org/10.1177/1753193410364484.
5. Iorio ML, Masden DL, Higgins JP. Cutaneous angiosome territory of the medial femoral condyle osteocutaneous flap. J Hand Surg Am. 2012;37(05):1033–41.
6. Iorio ML, Masden DL, Higgins JP. The limits of medial femoral condyle corticoperiosteal flaps. J Hand Surg Am. 2011;36(10):1592–6. https://doi.org/10.1016/j.jhsa.2011.07.015.
7. Higgins JP. Vascularized medial femoral condyle flap reconstruction for osseous defects of the hand and wrist. Hand Clin. 2024;40(1):151–9. https://doi.org/10.1016/j.hcl.2023.06.003.
8. Higgins JP, Bürger HK. Osteochondral flaps from the distal femur: expanding applications, harvest sites, and indications. J Reconstr Microsurg. 2014;30(7):483–90.
9. Pelzer M, Reichenberger M, Germann G. Osteo-periosteal-cutaneous flaps of the medial femoral condyle: a valuable modification for selected clinical situations. J Reconstr Microsurg. 2010;26(5):291–4. https://doi.org/10.1055/s-0030-1248239.
10. Miles MR, Jacobson L, Hill JB, Higgins JP, Giladi AM, Pet MA. Patient-reported lower extremity outcomes following fibula or medial femoral condyle free flaps for upper extremity defects. Hand (N Y). 2022:15589447211073827. https://doi.org/10.1177/15589447211073827.
11. Katz RD, Parks BG, Higgins JP. The axial stability of the femur after harvest of the medial femoral condyle corticocancellous flap: a biomechanical study of composite femur models. Microsurgery. 2012;32:213–8.
12. Endara MR, Brown BJ, Shuck J, Bachabi M, Parks BG, Higgins JP. Torsional stability of the femur after harvest of the medial femoral condyle corticocancellous flap. J Reconstr Microsurg. 2015;31:364–8.
13. Rao SS, Sexton CC, Higgins JP. Medial femoral condyle flap donor-site morbidity: a radiographic assessment. Plast Reconstr Surg. 2013;131(3):357e–62e.
14. Wong VW, Bürger HK, Iorio ML, Higgins JP. Lateral femoral condyle flap: an alternative source of vascularized bone from the distal femur. J Hand Surg Am. 2015;40(10):1972–80. https://doi.org/10.1016/j.jhsa.2015.06.106.
15. Wong VW, Higgins JP. Distally based iliotibial band flap: anatomic study with surgical considerations. J Reconstr Microsurg. 2016;32(7):551–5. https://doi.org/10.1055/s-0036-1583278.
16. Irwin CS, Higgins JP. Lateral femoral condyle flap. In: Chung KC, editor. Moran SL. ASSH surgical anatomy: flap reconstruction of the upper extremity; 2018. p. 296–300.
17. Garretson RB 3rd, Katolik LI, Verma N, Beck PR, Bach BR, Cole BJ. Contact pressure at osteochondral donor sites in the patellofemoral joint. Am J Sports Med. 2004;32(4):967–74. https://doi.org/10.1177/0363546503261706.
18. Burger HK, Windhofer C, Gaggl AJ, Higgins JP. Vascularized medial femoral trochlea osteocartilaginous flap reconstruction of proximal pole scaphoid nonunions. J Hand Surg Am. 2013;38(4):690–700. https://doi.org/10.1016/j.jhsa.2013.01.036.
19. Pet MA, Assi PE, Yousaf IS, Giladi AM, Higgins JP. Outcomes of the medial femoral trochlea Osteochondral free flap for proximal scaphoid reconstruction. J Hand Surg Am. 2020;45(4):317–26. e3. https://doi.org/10.1016/j.jhsa.2019.08.008.
20. Catapano J, Higgins JP. An algorithmic approach to the treatment of Kienbock disease. Hand Clin. 2022;38(4):417–24. https://doi.org/10.1016/j.hcl.2022.03.005.

21. Higgins JP, Burger H. Osteochondral free flap reconstruction of advanced Kienböck's disease. In: Lichtman D, Bain G, editors. Kienböck's disease: advances in diagnosis and treatment. Springer; 2016.
22. Pet MA, Assi PE, Giladi AM, Higgins JP. Preliminary clinical, radiographic, and patient-reported outcomes of the medial femoral trochlea Osteochondral free flap for lunate reconstruction in advanced Kienbock disease. J Hand Surg Am. 2020;45(8):774:e1-774 e8. https://doi.org/10.1016/j.jhsa.2019.12.008.
23. Burger HK, Windhofer C, Gaggl AJ, Higgins JP. Vascularized medial femoral trochlea osteochondral flap reconstruction of advanced Kienbock disease. J Hand Surg Am. 2014;39(7):1313–22. https://doi.org/10.1016/j.jhsa.2014.03.040.
24. Windhofer CM, Anoshina M, Ivusits P, Bürger HP. The free vascularized lateral femoral trochlea osteochondral graft: a reliable alternative for stage III Kienböck's disease. J Hand Surg Eur. 2021;46(10):1032–41.
25. Wong VW, Higgins JP. Medial femoral condyle flap. Plast Reconstr Surg Glob Open. 2016;4(8):e834. https://doi.org/10.1097/GOX.0000000000000815.
26. Pulos N, Kollitz KM, Bishop AT, Shin AY. Free vascularized medial femoral condyle bone graft after failed scaphoid nonunion surgery. J Bone Joint Surg Am. 2018;100(16):1379–86. https://doi.org/10.2106/JBJS.17.00955.
27. Doi K, Oda T, Soo-Heong T, Nanda V. Free vascularized bone graft for nonunion of the scaphoid. J Hand Surg Am. 2000;25(3):507–19. https://doi.org/10.1053/jhsu.2000.5993.
28. Higgins JP. Recalcitrant scaphoid proximal pole nonunion reconstructed with medial femoral condyle Osteoarticular graft. In: Yao J, editor. Scaphoid fractures and nonunions: a clinical casebook. Springer; 2015. p. 225–36.
29. Higgins JP, Sgromolo N. Avascular necrosis of the carpus. Hand surgery update VII. American Society for Surgery of the Hand; 2022.
30. Higgins JP, Burger HK. Proximal scaphoid arthroplasty using the medial femoral trochlea flap. J Wrist Surg. 2013;2(3):228–33. https://doi.org/10.1055/s-0033-1351789.
31. Daruwalla JH, Skrok J, Pet MA, Giladi AM, Higgins JP. Magnetic resonance imaging to investigate the clinical applicability of the medial femoral trochlea osteochondral flap within the wrist. Hand (N Y). 2022:15589447211064363. https://doi.org/10.1177/15589447211064363.
32. Van Handel AC, Lynch LM, Daruwalla JH, Higgins JP, Allen KL, Pet MA. Medial femoral trochlea flap reconstruction versus proximal row carpectomy for Kienbock's disease: a morphometric comparison. J Hand Surg Eur. 2021;46(10):1042–8. https://doi.org/10.1177/17531934211031862.
33. Windhofer CM, Higgins JP, Gaggl A, Burger HP. Lateral femoral trochlea Osteochondral flap reconstruction of proximal pole scaphoid nonunions. J Hand Surg Am. 2022; https://doi.org/10.1016/j.jhsa.2022.08.019.
34. Pet MA, Higgins JP. Long-term outcomes of vascularized trochlear flaps for scaphoid proximal pole reconstruction. Hand Clin. 2019;35(3):345–52. https://doi.org/10.1016/j.hcl.2019.03.006.
35. Anoshina M, Higgins JP, Jiga L, Burger H. Treatment of Kienböck's disease using free vascularized cartilage bone flaps from the lateral femoral condyle. In: Gravvanis A, Kakagia DD, Ramakrishnan V, editors. Clinical scenarios in reconstructive microsurgery. Springer; 2022.
36. Higgins JP, Guarino GM, Belyea CM, Tintle SM. Lateral femoral trochlea flap reconstruction of the proximal capitate: an assessment of congruity and description of technique. J Hand Surg Am. 2023;48(2):149–57. https://doi.org/10.1016/j.jhsa.2022.04.015.
37. Miles MR, Higgins JP. Scaphoid nonunion: medial femoral condyle vascularized bone graft. In: Beredjiklian PK, Matzon JL, editors. Hand surgery-tricks of the trade. Thieme; 2020.
38. Assi P, Giladi AM, Higgins JP. Free vascularized medial femoral condyle grafts for reconstruction of nonunions and avascular necrosis in the hand and wrist. In: Huang JI, Hunt DR, editors. Operative techniques in orthopaedic surgery. Wolters Kluwer; 2021.
39. Higgins JP, Burger HK. Medial femoral trochlea Osteochondral flap: applications for scaphoid and lunate reconstruction. Clin Plast Surg. 2017;44(2):257–65. https://doi.org/10.1016/j.cps.2016.11.004.

40. Higgins JP, Burger HK. Medial femoral trochlea osteochondral flap: applications for scaphoid and lunate reconstruction. Clin Plast Surg. 2020;47(4):491–9. https://doi.org/10.1016/j.cps.2020.06.004.
41. Higgins JP, Bürger HK. The use of osteochondral flaps in the treatment of carpal disorders. J Hand Surg Eur. 2018;43(1):48–56. https://doi.org/10.1177/1753193417739545.

Chapter 4
Osteocutaneous Radial Forearm Free Flap

Sarah M. Drejet and Jason P. Hunt

Introduction

The osteocutaneous radial forearm free flap (OCRFFF) is a variation of the more commonly used radial forearm free flap (RFFF) that involves harvesting partial thickness of the radius just proximal to the radial flare in addition to a skin paddle. The radial forearm free flap was first used and described by Dr. Yang and Dr. Gao at the Shenyang Military Hospital in 1978 [21]. This led to the rise of the use of the OCRFFF in the early 1980s followed by its decline in use in the late 1980s due to significant donor site morbidities, primarily fracture of the forearm [13, 15, 16]. It has been described in its reconstruction of midface [1] and mandibular defects [2], but also of foot and ankle reconstruction and lower extremity defects [4], hand reconstruction [20], and phalloplasty [8]. Historically, its use has been limited due to the concern for radius fracture, but this risk has become a rare event with the implementation of prophylactic plating of the radius [18]. Alternatives to its use in midface and mandibular reconstruction include the osteocutaneous iliac crest, scapular, and fibular free flaps.

Indications

The OCRFFF is most commonly used in mandible and midface head and neck reconstructions. It is a very versatile flap due to the advantages of having a long vascular pedicle, pliable skin and soft tissue, and reliable vascular anatomy.

S. M. Drejet (✉) · J. P. Hunt
Department of Otolaryngology – Head and Neck Surgery, University of Utah School of Medicine, Salt Lake City, UT, USA
e-mail: sarah.drejet@hci.utah.edu

J. P. Agarwal, D. W. Mathes (eds.), *Bone Flaps in Reconstructive Surgery*,
https://doi.org/10.1007/978-3-032-12540-8_4

Though dental implants have been performed [6] in the OCRFFF, it is mostly felt to have insufficient bone stock for placement of dental implants. However, there may be an evolving role for implants with the use of bone grafts and bone morphogenetic protein-2 products [17]. Additionally, the length of bone that can be harvested ranges up to 14 cm and osteotomies of the harvested bone can be successfully performed [12]. It is critical to maintain the periosteum and a minimum of 2.5-cm segments to preserve the blood supply to the bone [12]. This reconstruction is contraindicated in patients with a dominant radial artery and/or lack of collateral blood flow between the palmar arches. Caution should be exercised in using this flap in patients with prior traumatic injury or fracture of the forearm.

Pertinent Anatomy

The OCRFFF is supplied by the radial artery, with venous drainage via the vena comitantes and/or cephalic vein. In the forearm, the radial and ulnar arteries branch off of the brachial artery at the antecubital fossa and together they give blood supply to the hand via the deep and superficial palmar arches respectively. These arches are connected to create collateral flow to the hand. It is essential to ensure sufficient collateral blood flow to the hand before harvesting the radial artery. Failure to do so can result in ischemic damage to the hand [5].

Numerous techniques have been reported for testing collateral blood flow in the forearm [7, 11, 19]. The simplest of these is to perform a subjective Allen test. This is done by occluding the ulnar and radial arteries at the wrist, having the patient pump their fist and elevate their hand to drain the blood and then release only the ulnar artery to ensure good capillary refill returns to the entire hand while the radial artery remains occluded. If this test is inconclusive, the collateral flow can also be confirmed by using a handheld Doppler on the palmar arches or a pulse oximeter on the thumb or index finger and repeating the steps of the Allen test. If Doppler signal returns or if the pulse oximeter is not dampened or delayed in its return, this is confirmation of intact collateral flow. If none of these studies conclusively demonstrates good blood flow, an arterial duplex or a computer tomography angiography (CTA) can be performed of the upper extremity. If collateral blood supply cannot be confirmed, an alternative flap should be considered.

The venous drainage of the OCRFF is via a deep system of vena comitantes that run in parallel with the radial artery deep to the brachioradialis between the brachioradialis and flexor carpi radialis and a superficial system of the cephalic vein that runs over the brachioradialis. In the majority of patients, these deep and superficial systems connect at the antecubital fossa via the anterior perforating vein [10] and allow for the option of either connecting one vein or splitting the superficial and deep systems from each other. The average venous pedicle length is 14–22 cm, depending highly on the length of the forearm and size of skin paddle to be harvested [3].

Two nerves are typically encountered during the harvest of the OCRFFF. One is the superficial radial nerve which runs deep to the brachioradialis until it emerges superficially through a split in the brachioradialis tendon within the distal forearm. This nerve should be identified and preserved to maintain sensation of the radial aspect of the dorsal hand. The other is the lateral antebrachial cutaneous nerve which is typically transected and is of minimal consequence as it gives sensation to the portion of skin being harvested. It can be harvested if a sensate flap is desired.

The skin paddle for the flap is centered over the distal third of the radial artery, where the artery travels between the brachioradialis tendon and the flexor carpi radialis tendon. Large skin paddles can be harvested but this is limited by the need to maintain some lymphatic drainage from the hand. Harvesting skin paddles up to 30 cm in length and 15 cm in width while maintaining a 3–5-cm strip of skin on the dorsal surface of the forearm has been described.

The fasciocutaneous perforators extend from the pedicle to the skin paddle in the distal one-third of the forearm between the brachioradialis and flexor carpi radialis.

The periosteal feeding vessels lie within the lateral intramuscular septum just deep to the brachioradialis tendon and it is important not to disrupt them to maintain vascularity of the bone.

Along the radial surface of the radius there are muscular attachments of the brachioradialis along the distal end. The volar surface of the radius serves as an insertion point for the pronator quadratus, the flexor digitorum superficialis, and flexor pollicis. The flexor digitorum superficialis and flexor pollicis also frequently interdigitate more superficially along the radial artery itself. These all must be released to free the harvested portion of cortical bone with the fasciocutaneous skin paddle. If more than 7 cm of bone is to be harvested, then the pronator teres muscle will also need to be released from the radius and resuspended after harvest.

The radius is a spiral-shaped bone from which only a portion of the thickness can be harvested. Up to 14 cm in length of cortical bone can be harvested from the radius and one to two osteotomies can be performed in the harvested bone safely. Most will strive to harvest 50% of the cross section of the bone and this will typically yield an average width of bone of about 1.0–1.3 cm [17]. Prior to the implementation of prophylactic plating, radius fracture rates following OCRFFF harvest ranged from 8% to 67%, with an average of 24% [18]. This prompted two studies evaluating bone strength. One reported that osteotomized formalin-fixed human radii were only 24% as strong as intact radii [14] and the other, which evaluated osteotomized sheep tibia, reported they were only 15–28% as strong as intact bones [9]. Since the implementation of prophylactic plating, fracture rates have dropped significantly with Werle et al. reporting no clinically significant radius fractures in 52 patients and serial radiographs demonstrating remodeling and reconstitution of the donor radii without localized osteopenia [18].

Harvest Technique of the Osteocutaneous Radial Forearm Free Flap

Preparation

This flap is typically harvested under general anesthesia. The entire arm or lower arm may be prepped, according to the surgeon's preference, and the arm is placed on an arm board. One of the major benefits of using the forearm as a donor site for the head and neck or lower extremity is the ability to harvest while simultaneously preparing or managing the recipient site. Many surgeons prefer to harvest the forearm free flap under tourniquet. A pressure of 250 mm Hg is used on a tourniquet around the bicep using a size-appropriate tourniquet for the patient. Prior to inflation of the tourniquet some surgeons may choose to exsanguinate the arm with an Esmarch bandage. Regardless, the tourniquet should be maintained for no more than 2 h.

Design

In designing the skin paddle and its location on the forearm, it is important to preserve the distal forearm skin over the styloid process to minimize the risk of hardware exposure. Compared to the fasciocutaneous RFFF, this skin paddle should be moved 1–2 cm proximally up the forearm. Alternatively, the pronator quadratus muscle and flexor pollicis longus muscle can be used to help cover the distal plate. Similar to a RFFF, the skin paddle is centered along the radial artery and, as shown in Fig. 4.1, is often designed to incorporate the cephalic vein. A lazy-S incision is then extended from the forearm skin paddle up to the antebrachial crease with a back cut to prevent scar contracture through the crease.

Incisions are then made around the skin paddle down through skin and subcutaneous tissue to expose the fascia overlying the forearm muscles. Ulnarly, the flexor carpi radialis and the palmaris longus tendons are identified. Dissection can

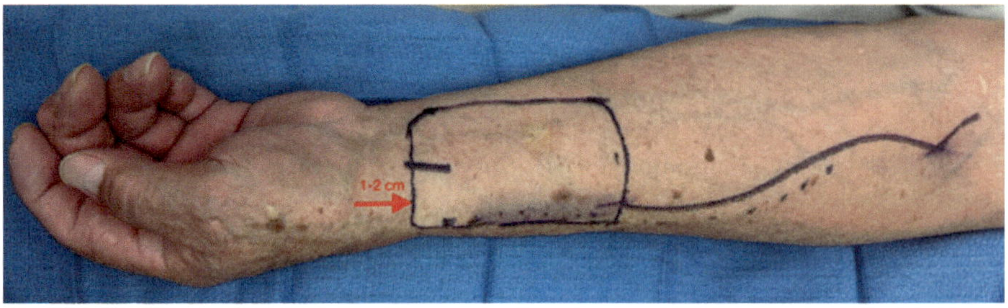

Fig. 4.1 This photograph shows a possible flap design at a location 1–2 cm proximal to the wrist crease and also proximal to the palpable landmark of the styloid process

be carried out subfascial or suprafascial until the muscle belly of the FCR is encountered. Radially, the brachioradialis fascia is identified and preserved to the ulnar edge of the tendon. The radial nerve and cephalic vein are encountered here running longitudinally along the brachioradialis. The cephalic vein is harvested with the flap to maintain a second venous drainage system and is often dissected into the antecubital fossa where it can be harvested as a single venous outflow with contributions from vena comitantes and the cephalic vein. Care must be taken to identify the superficial radial nerve where it exits a split in the brachioradialis tendon.

The ulnar edge of the brachioradialis tendon is identified and undermined. Sharp dissection is used here to closely approximate the brachioradialis tendon to preserve perforators extending from the radial artery to the bone as shown in Fig. 4.2. The brachioradialis is separated from the underlying fascia until the radial aspect of the brachioradialis tendon is identified distally and can be retracted radially. More proximally, this dissection is carried subfascially where the radial nerve courses deep to the brachioradialis tendon. Distally, the brachioradialis tendon can also be sharply dissected off of the radial flare to allow improved exposure for bony cuts and plating. In order to do this, the distal end of the cephalic vein is transected and the distal radial nerve is dissected free from the flap and retracted radially with the brachioradialis tendon.

The radial aspect of the dissection is extended down to the muscle bellies of the flexor digitorum superficialis and flexor pollicis. The muscles attach to the pedicle itself but also to the radial surface of the radius. These muscles can be gently retracted to determine their end action and differentiate the two (moving either the thumb alone or all fingers with applied tension). These muscles are then released from the pedicle and the portion of bone to be harvested. A small cuff of muscle can be taken to avoid compromising the vascular supply to the bone. These steps for managing the musculature can be seen in Figs. 4.3, 4.4, and 4.5.

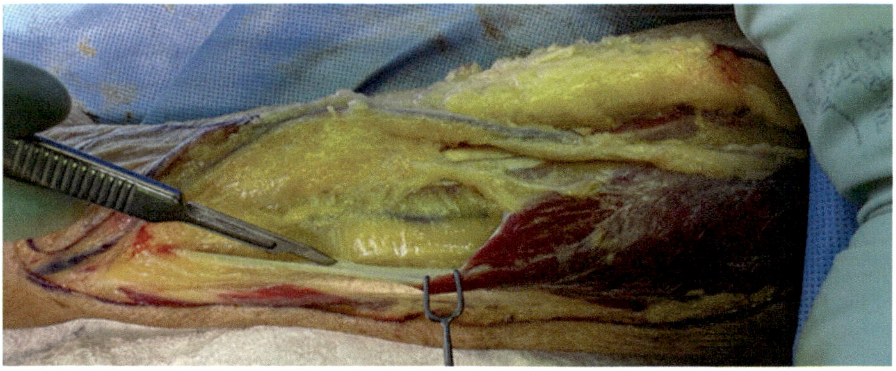

Fig. 4.2 The photograph shows a knife being used to execute sharp dissection along the brachioradialis tendon to preserve perforators extending from the radial artery to the bone. The cephalic vein is pulled towards the ulnar side of the arm together with the skin paddle. Also visible in the photograph is the deep aspect of the radial nerve where it courses underneath the brachioradialis tendon

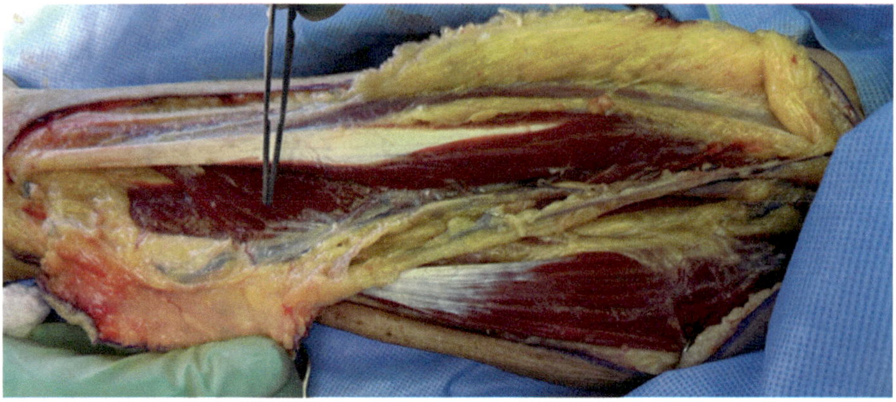

Fig. 4.3 In this photograph the pedicle and skin paddle are gently retracted towards the radial aspect of the arm. The instrument points to the muscle belly of the flexor digitorum superficialis and more distally the flexor pollicis can be seen. These will both be released in the harvest of the OCRFFF. Small branches, seen extending from the pedicle to the muscle bellies, must also be ligated and transected

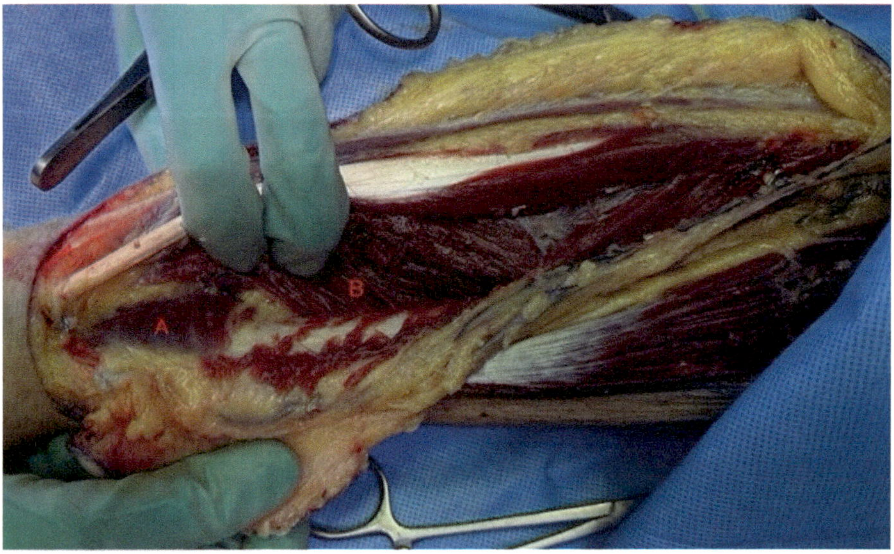

Fig. 4.4 In this photograph the skin paddle is being retracted towards the radial aspect of the arm. The fllexor digitorum superficialis and flexor pollicis have been released and the broad attachment of the pronator quadratus can be seen coursing transversely across the distal radius. A, pronator quadratus; B, flexor digitorum superficialis and flexor pollicis

Once the flexor digitorum superficialis and flexor pollicis muscles have been released, then the pronator quadratus can be identified with its broad attachment transversely across the distal radius. The pronator quadratus is then transected at the approximate 50% cross-sectional line of the radius in preparation for the bony harvest.

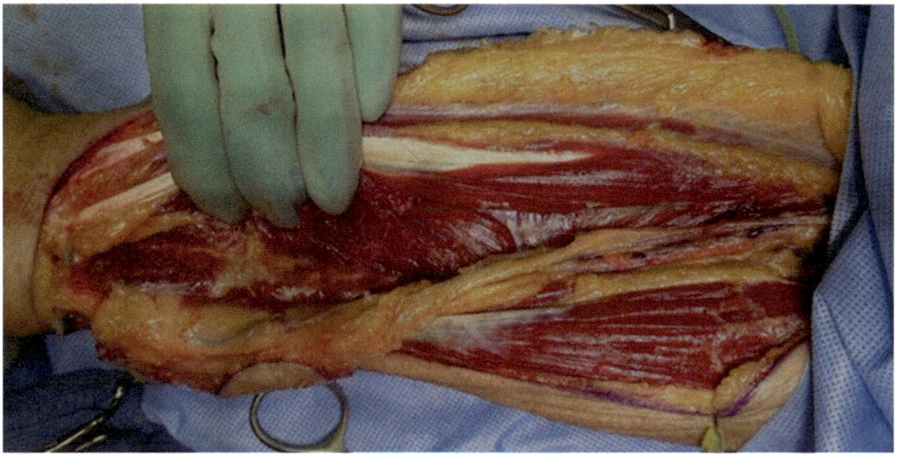

Fig. 4.5 A photograph with the skin paddle retracted towards the radial aspect of the arm shows the pronator quadratus has been transected at approximately the 50% line of the radius. This allows for bone cuts to harvest approximately 50% of the cross section of the bone

Typically, osteotomies are made ulnarly with a sagittal saw and then distally, followed by the radial and proximal osteotomies. With the forearm supinated, the first longitudinal bone osteotomy along the ulnar surface is made with a sagittal saw using either a finger or instrument to confirm the full width of the radius and ensure approximately 50% is being harvested. Proximal and distal osteotomies are made in a neutral handshake position and the radial osteotomy is made with the hand pronated by an assistant. This helps accommodate the spiral nature of the bone. The distal osteotomy is made just proximal to the flare of the radius to allow for a distal radius fracture plate to be used. It is essential not to past cut at the proximal and distal ends as this can significantly weaken the remaining bone. Many surgeons favor a boat-shaped osteotomy with bevels at the ends and this may minimize past cutting. However, with prophylactic plating there is less evidence of this being necessary. If greater than 6–7 cm of bone is needed, the pronator teres will need to be released. This should be resuspended after prophylactic plating has been performed. The steps for performing the bone cuts can be seen in Figs. 4.6, 4.7, 4.8, and 4.9. Prophylactic plating can occur via a dorsal or volar method. The volar method as shown in Fig. 4.10 has the advantage of easier coverage with muscle that will decrease the risk of plate exposure. The authors collaborate with hand specialists to perform the prophylactic plating.

After the plating is performed, the flexor muscles are approximated to the brachioradialis to provide plate coverage as shown in Fig. 4.11. A split thickness skin graft is typically harvested and applied to the muscle for skin coverage. The final result at 2 weeks can be seen in Fig. 4.12.

Figures 4.13, 4.14, 4.15, 4.16, 4.17, and 4.18 show the technique being used for a midface reconstruction following a maxillectomy for cancer with early results. Long-term results in a different patient can be seen in Figs. 4.19 and 4.20. It should be noted that while dental implants remain challenging, there are other options for

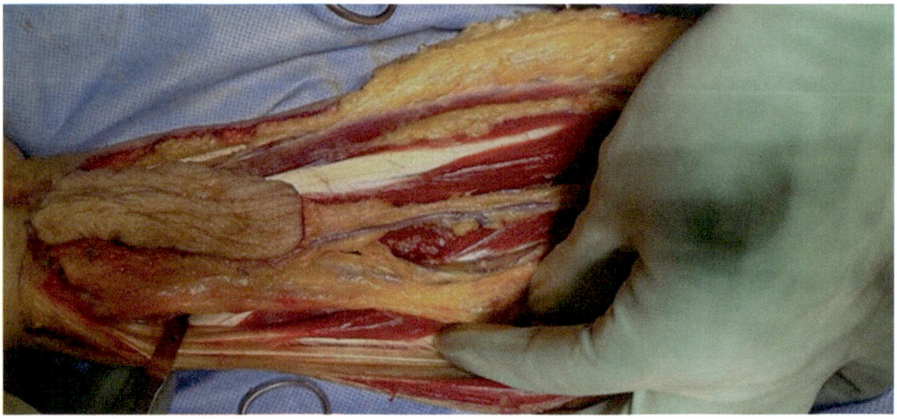

Fig. 4.6 This photograph shows the tendon of the branchioradialis muscle being retracted radially together with the extensor muscles to allow access for planning and making the bony cuts

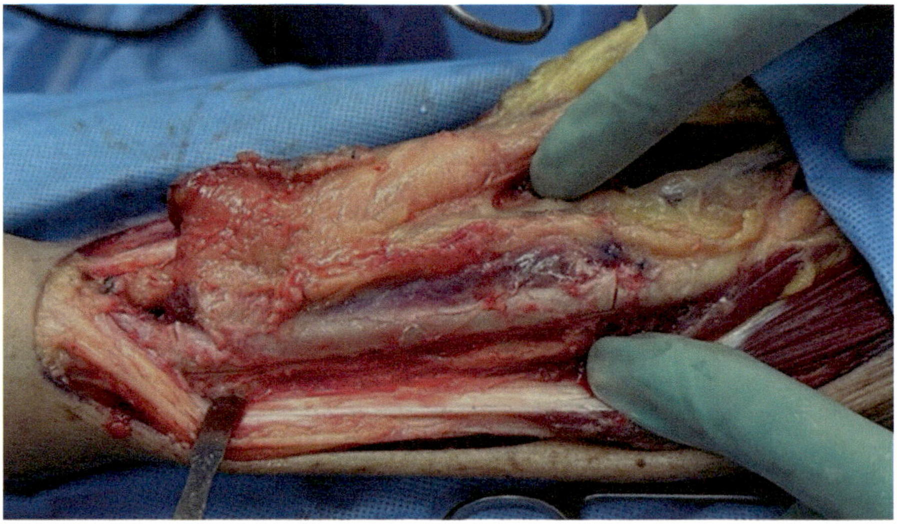

Fig. 4.7 This is a photograph of the radius bone from the radial side. Bone cuts are made. Approximately 50% of the cross section of the bone has been harvested

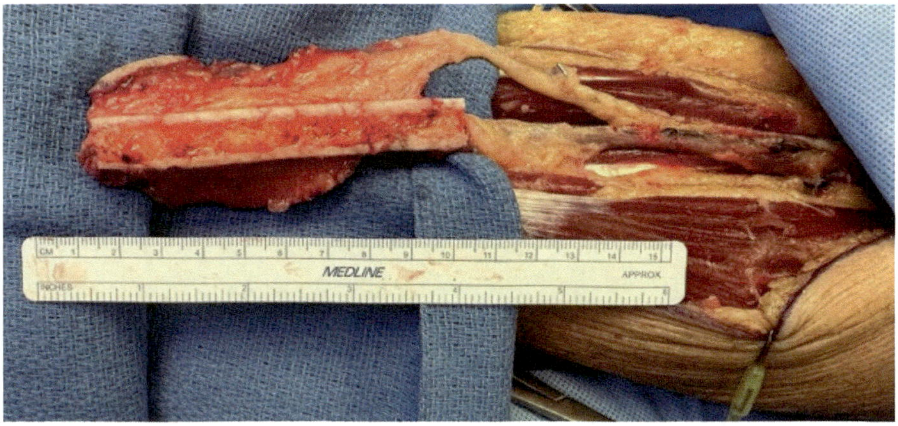

Fig. 4.8 This is a photograph of the OCRFFF still attached to the forearm via the vascular pedicle. An 8.5-cm length of bone with skin paddle attached and lying underneath it can be seen

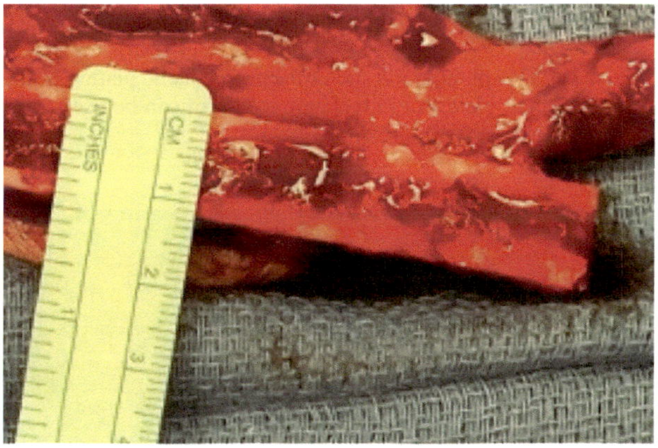

Fig. 4.9 This is a close up photograph of the harvested bone. The cross-sectional area of bone is 1.2cm. The bone appears to be well perfused with bleeding from the marrow space

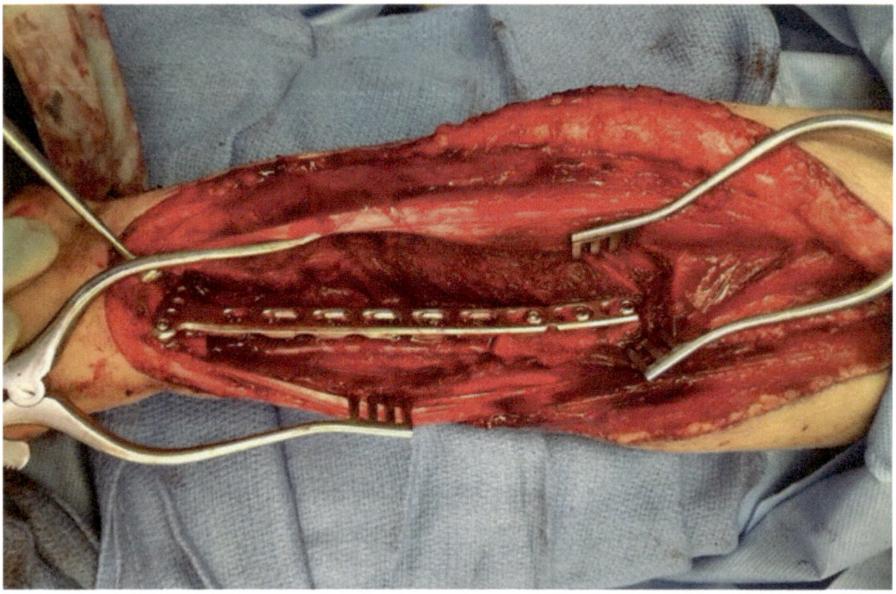

Fig. 4.10 This photograph shows the prophylactic plating of the volar surface of the radius with a mini-fragment plate. An intraoperative C-arm can be used to ensure bicortical screws are placed without causing functional impairment

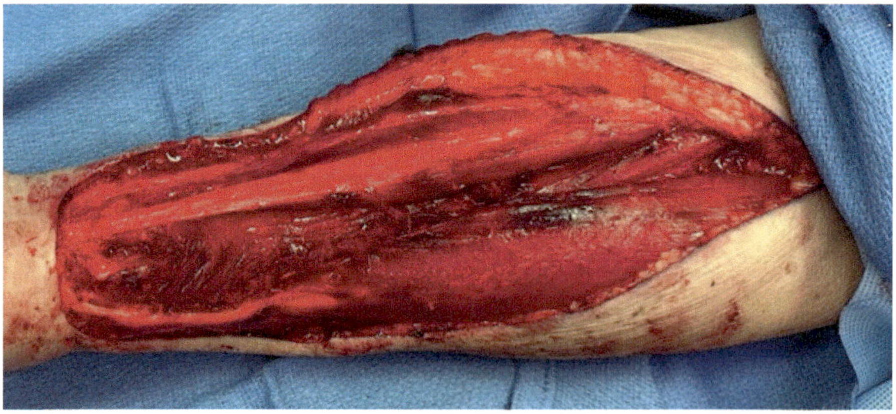

Fig. 4.11 This photograph shows a the mini fragment plate now covered by muscle. Coverage of the plate accomplished by advancing flexor muscles over the plate and securing them to the brachioradialis tendon. Care is taken to preserve the radial nerve

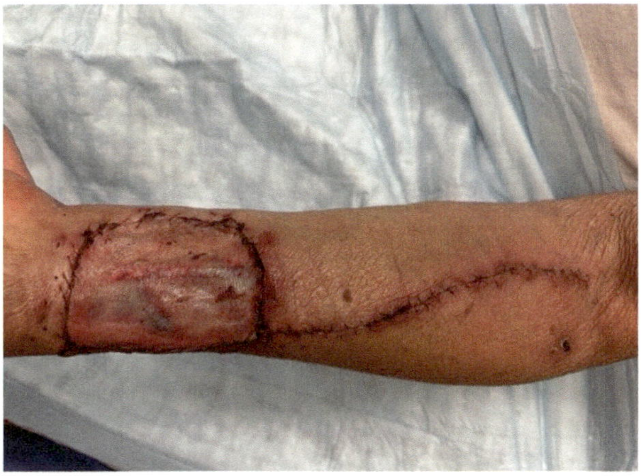

Fig. 4.12 A photograph taken two weeks after surgery shows the forearm is healing appropriately without any tendon or plate exposure

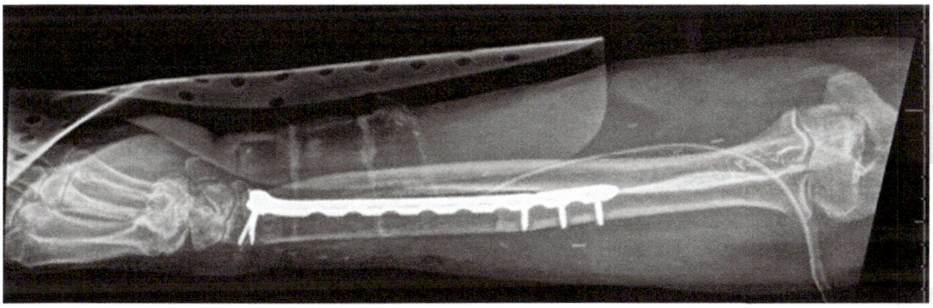

Fig. 4.13 Lateral X-ray of the forearm demonstrates the placement of the mini-fragment prophylactic forearm plate. The externally placed forearm splint is also captured

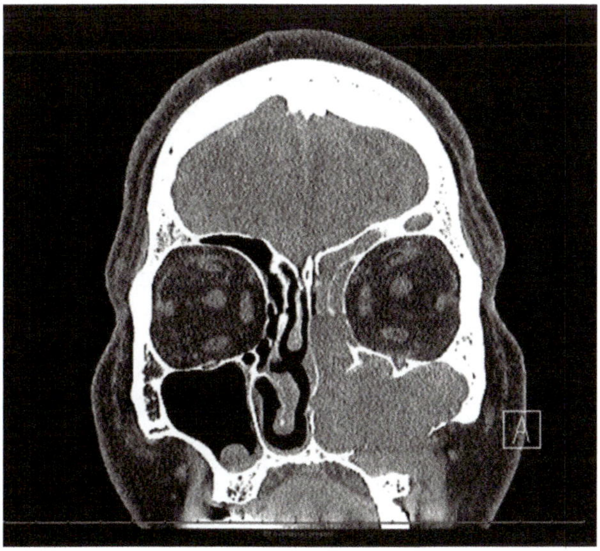

Fig. 4.14 A coronal CT scan demonstrates tumor eroding through the lateral wall of the maxilla indicating the need for maxillectomy

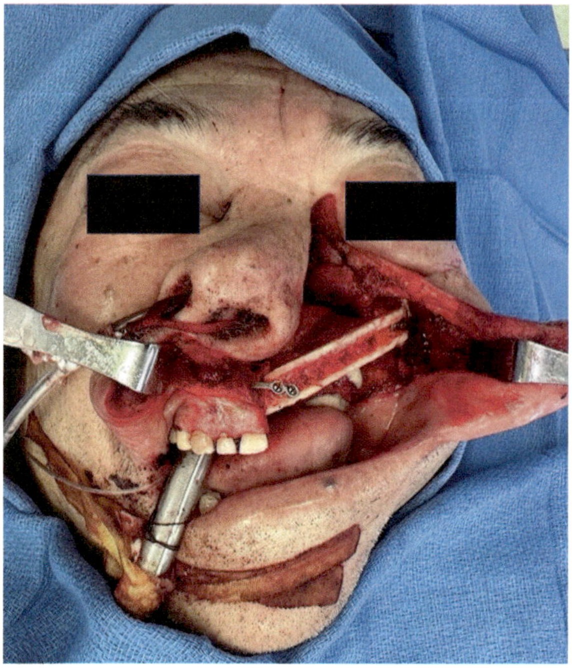

Fig. 4.15 An intraoperative photograph shows the bony inset of a radial forearm. The bone is cut to size and the marrow side is plated to the remnant maxillary alveolus and zygoma with mini midface plates. This helps maintain the projection of the midface

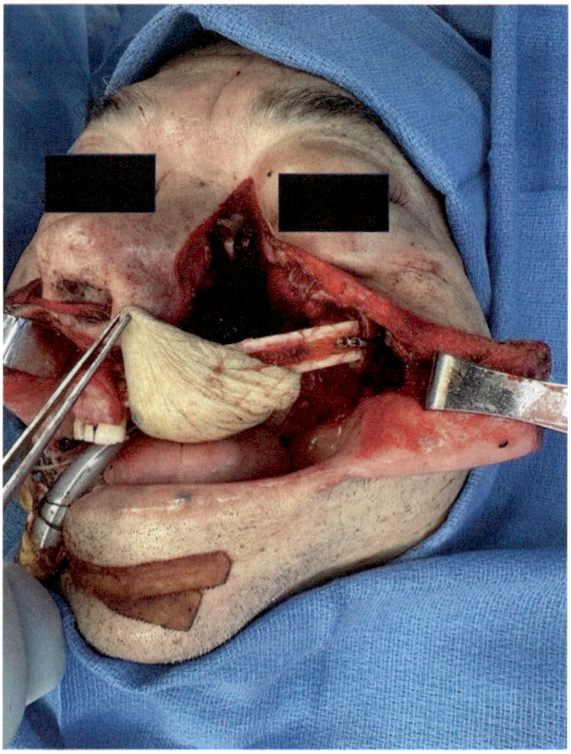

Fig. 4.16 An intraoperative photograph shows the forearm bone secured in place with mini midface plates and a pick-up holding the skin paddle is used to demonstrate its mobility for reconstructing the inner lining of the roof of the mouth

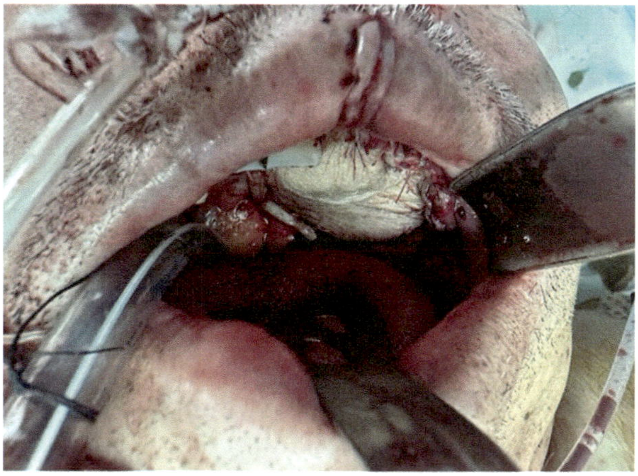

Fig. 4.17 An intraoperative intraoral photograph demonstrates the soft tissue inset of the forearm skin paddle into the oral cavity defect, as well as the primary closure of the lip

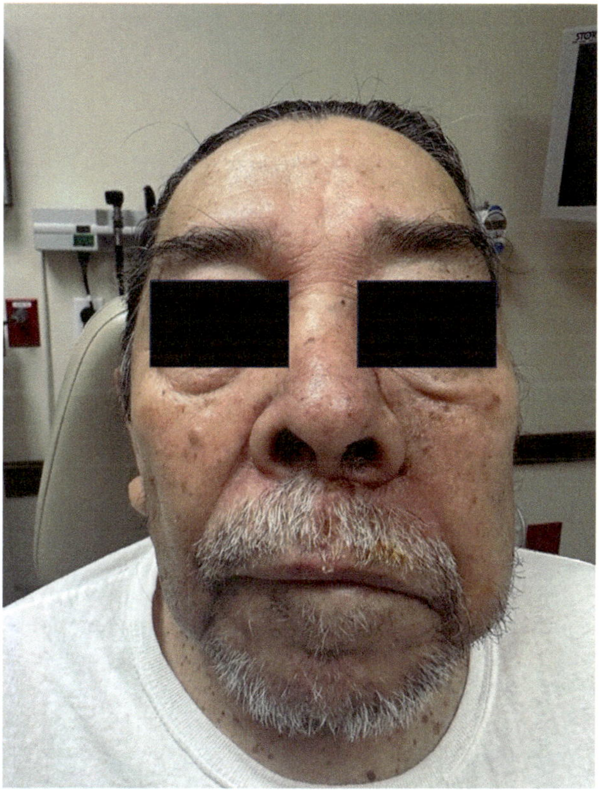

Fig. 4.18 A photograph taken of the patient two-weeks after surgery shows maintenance of midface projection. There is some residual droop of the left midface soft tissues from release of the musculature from the maxilla during resection

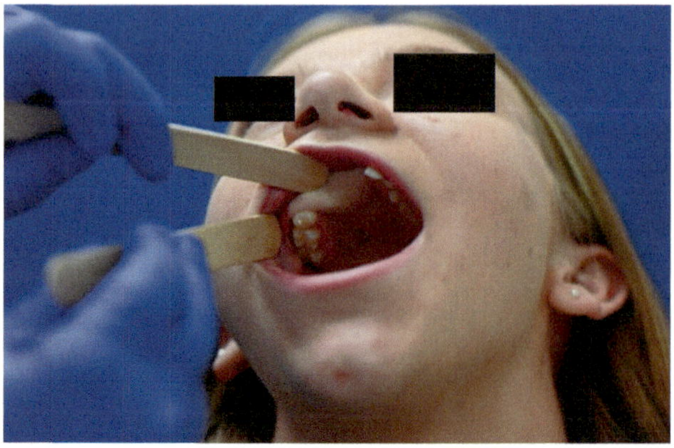

Fig. 4.19 A photograph of the patient's intraoral examination shows the skin paddle of the OCRFFF well incorporated into the oral cavity

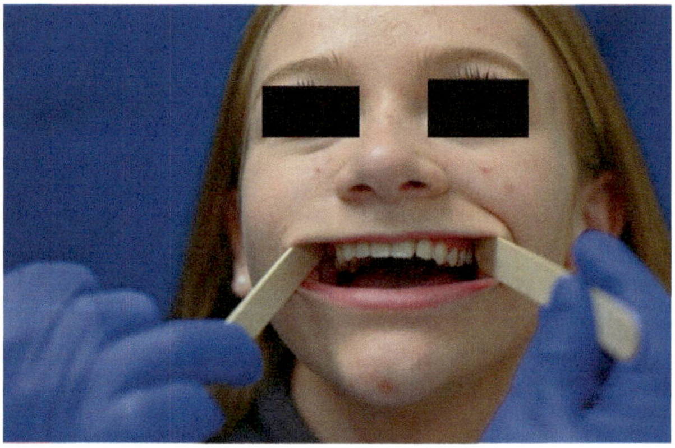

Fig. 4.20 A photograph of the patient shows a partial denture in place over the right maxillary alveolar reconstruction

dental restoration including dental bridges and partial dentures. With a pliable skin paddle, these restorations can be accomplished more easily than with some other osteocutaneous alternatives.

Case 1: Patient Requiring Infrastructure Maxillectomy with Orbital Preservation for Squamous Cell Carcinoma of the Left Maxilla

Case 2: Pediatric Patient Requiring Limited Infrastructure Maxillectomy for Epithelial sarcoma of the Maxilla, Reconstructed with a OCRFFF at the Age of 13, Now Photographed at 17 Years Old

Summary

- OCRFFF is a reliable reconstructive option for midface and mandibular reconstruction.
- Advantages include long pedicle, pliable skin and soft tissue, and reliable vascular anatomy.

- Disadvantages include limited bony stock for dental implants and limited bone length (up to 14 cm).
- With prophylactic plating of the forearm, OCRFFF has similar complication rates with other head and neck bony reconstructive options.

References

1. Ahmad FI, Means C, Labby AB, Troob SH, Gonzalez JD, Kim MM, et al. Osteocutaneous radial forearm free flap in nonmandible head and neck reconstruction. Head Neck. 2017;39(9):1888–93. https://doi.org/10.1002/hed.24863.
2. Arganbright JM, Tsue TT, Girod DA, Militsakh ON, Sykes KJ, Markey J, Shnayder Y. Outcomes of the osteocutaneous radial forearm free flap for mandibular reconstruction. JAMA Otolaryngol Head Neck Surg. 2013;139(2):168–72. https://doi.org/10.1001/jamaoto.2013.1615.
3. Bigcas J-LM., Bond J. Osteocutaneous radial forearm flap in NBK564384. 2024.
4. Capito AE, Hansen BK, Schmitt MW, Beck JH, Cripe BA, Apel PJ. Osteocutaneous radial forearm flap: harvest technique and prophylactic volar locked plating. Plast Reconstr Surg Glob Open. 2023;11(11):e5449. https://doi.org/10.1097/GOX.0000000000005449.
5. Chim H, Bakri K, Moran SL. Complications related to radial artery occlusion, radial artery harvest, and arterial lines. Hand Clin. 2015;31(1):93–100. https://doi.org/10.1016/j.hcl.2014.09.010.
6. Gonzalez-Castro J, Petrisor D, Ballard D, Wax MK. The double-barreled radial forearm osteocutaneous free flap. Laryngoscope. 2016;126(2):340–4. https://doi.org/10.1002/lary.25388.
7. Khan AS, Henton JM, Adams TS, Dwivedi RC, Harris PA. Evaluation of hand circulation before radial forearm free flap surgery. Laryngoscope. 2009;119(9):1679–81. https://doi.org/10.1002/lary.20556.
8. Kim SK, Lee KC, Kwon YS, Cha BH. Phalloplasty using radial forearm osteocutaneous free flaps in female-to-male transsexuals. J Plast Reconstr Aesthet Surg. 2009;62(3):309–17. https://doi.org/10.1016/j.bjps.2007.11.011.
9. Meland NB, Maki S, Chao EY, Rademaker B. The radial forearm flap: a biomechanical study of donor-site morbidity utilizing sheep tibia. Plast Reconstr Surg. 1992;90(5):763–73.
10. Moreno MA, Small LT, Gardner JR, Kim AH, Vural E, Sunde J. Outcomes of single anastomoses for superficial and deep-system venous drainage of radial forearm free flaps. OTO Open. 2021;5(2):2473974X211006927. https://doi.org/10.1177/2473974X211006927.
11. Nuckols DA, Tsue TT, Toby EB, Girod DA. Preoperative evaluation of the radial forearm free flap patient with the objective Allen's test. Otolaryngol Head Neck Surg. 2000;123(5):553–7. https://doi.org/10.1067/mhn.2000.110728.
12. Silverman DA, Przylecki WH, Arganbright JM, Shnayder Y, Kakarala K, Nazir N, et al. Evaluation of bone length and number of osteotomies utilizing the osteocutaneous radial forearm free flap for mandible reconstruction: an 8-year review of complications and flap survival. Head Neck. 2016;38(3):434–8. https://doi.org/10.1002/hed.23919.
13. Soutar DS, McGregor IA. The radial forearm flap in intraoral reconstruction: the experience of 60 consecutive cases. Plast Reconstr Surg. 1986;78(1):1–8. https://doi.org/10.1097/00006534-198607000-00001.
14. Swanson E, Boyd JB, Mulholland RS. The radial forearm flap: a biomechanical study of the osteotomized radius. Plast Reconstr Surg. 1990;85(2):267–72.
15. Timmons MJ, Missotten FE, Poole MD, Davies DM. Complications of radial forearm flap donor sites. Br J Plast Surg. 1986;39(2):176–8. https://doi.org/10.1016/0007-1226(86)90078-0.
16. Vaughan ED. The radial forearm free flap in orofacial reconstruction. Personal experience in 120 consecutive cases. J Craniomaxillofac Surg. 1990;18(1):2–7. https://doi.org/10.1016/s1010-5182(05)80596-7.

17. Virgin FW, Iseli TA, Iseli CE, Sunde J, Carroll WR, Magnuson JS, Rosenthal EL. Functional outcomes of fibula and osteocutaneous forearm free flap reconstruction for segmental mandibular defects. Laryngoscope. 2010;120(4):663–7. https://doi.org/10.1002/lary.20791.
18. Werle AH, Tsue TT, Toby EB, Girod DA. Osteocutaneous radial forearm free flap: its use without significant donor site morbidity. Otolaryngol Head Neck Surg. 2000;123(6):711–7. https://doi.org/10.1067/mhn.2000.110865.
19. Wood JW, Broussard KC, Burkey B. Preoperative testing for radial forearm free flaps to reduce donor site morbidity. JAMA Otolaryngol Head Neck Surg. 2013;139(2):183–6. https://doi.org/10.1001/jamaoto.2013.1357.
20. Yajima H, Tamai S, Yamauchi T, Mizumoto S. Osteocutaneous radial forearm flap for hand reconstruction. J Hand Surg Am. 1999;24(3):594–603. https://doi.org/10.1053/jhsu.1999.0594.
21. Yang GF, Chen PJ, Gao YZ, Liu XY, Li J, Jiang SX, He SP. Forearm free skin flap transplantation: a report of 56 cases. 1981. Br J Plast Surg. 1997;50(3):162–5. https://doi.org/10.1016/s0007-1226(97)91363-1.

Chapter 5
Osteocutaneous Scapular Flaps

Danielle Olla and Evan Matros

Introduction

The free fibula flap is the most commonly performed flap for bony reconstruction. It is utilized to reconstruct defects in various parts of the body such as the head and neck, upper and lower extremities, spine, and pelvic regions [1–5]. However, in cases where performing a fibula flap is not possible due to contraindications like peripheral vascular disease (PVD), history of trauma, or prior use of fibula flaps, or in complex cases requiring additional significant soft tissue needs, other options should be considered. The scapular region has a variety of potential chimeric components from a single-source vessel which can include tissue types such as bone, muscle, fascia, and soft tissue. Hallock looked at the combinations of flaps from the major subscapular branches off the axillary artery and found over five dozen possible different arrangements. He discussed the advantages of these combined free flaps in his practice from 1982 to 1995. He used these chimeric flaps to augment surface area, protect microanastomoses, provide coverage of disparate sites, achieve gliding surfaces, create dynamic reanimation of multiple muscles, and assemble composite flaps including vascularized bone [6].

The description of the territory and concept of a bony flap based on the subscapular system was reported in 1978 by Saijo [7]. He described that the osseous portion of the conventional scapular flap was supplied by branches of the circumflex scapular artery. In 1982, Gilbert and Teot published their experience using the subscapular system in fasciocutaneous free flaps with two skin paddle designs called scapular

D. Olla
Moffitt Cancer Center, Tampa, FL, USA
e-mail: Danielle.Olla@Moffitt.org

E. Matros (✉)
Memorial Sloan Kettering Cancer Center, New York, NY, USA
e-mail: matrose@mskcc.org

J. P. Agarwal, D. W. Mathes (eds.), *Bone Flaps in Reconstructive Surgery*, https://doi.org/10.1007/978-3-032-12540-8_5

and parascapular flaps [8]. A few years later, Swartz et al. published their findings in eight cadavers and clinical experience with 26 patients with a reliable blood supply to the lateral border of the scapula based on branches of the circumflex scapular artery. They reported that the lateral border of the scapula provided up to 14 cm of thick, straight corticocancellous bone that could be osteotomized [9]. Coleman and Sultan published their results on 14 cadaveric and 22 operative dissections with an additional blood supply to the lower lateral boarder and the tip of the scapula arising from the thoracodorsal axis called the angular artery. They found it proximal or distal to the serratus branch of the thoracodorsal artery and then arborizing to the periosteum on the deep surface of the scapula tip. This discovery opened the door to two separate vascular pedicles for two bony segments from the scapula which they named the bipedicled osteocutaneous scapular flap [10]. Seneviratne et al. continued this research with anatomic studies to look specifically at the angular branch and anatomic variants. About half the time, they found the angular branch came off the thoracodorsal artery distal to the branch of the serratus anterior; 25% of the time it came off the serratus anterior branch itself; 20% there was a trifurcation of the serratus, thoracodorsal, and angular branches; and 4% of the time the angular branch came off proximal to the serratus branch [11].

Scapular bone has been well established as a safe reliable option for osseous reconstruction. A wide array of defects can be reconstructed including maxillary, mandibular, and calvarial defects. Hasan et al. published their work utilizing 42 scapular flaps in several combinations and defects. They presented an algorithm for lateral or anterior mandibular bone defects [12]. Depending on the defect, they proposed different options including one or both bony vascular pedicles (circumflex scapular and angular artery) and other tissue including muscle (teres major, latissimus dorsi) and soft tissue (parascapular). Of the 42 scapular flaps, they had 2 flap failures. Recently, a larger study of 208 scapular free flaps for mandibular reconstruction was published with excellent function and aesthetic outcomes. There were 7 microvascular thromboses, 5 cases of total flap necrosis, and 6 cases of scapular fracture [13].

Studies have compared the use of the fibula, iliac crest, and scapula for bony maxillofacial reconstruction. Wilkman et al. conducted a study and found that out of 92 deep circumflex iliac artery flaps (56%), 42 scapular flaps (26%), and 29 fibular flaps (18%), the highest rate of flap loss was observed in the deep circumflex iliac artery group. There were no significant differences in the number of early or late complications between the flaps, but donor site complications were more severe in the iliac crest group. Dental implants and osteotomies were performed safely in all groups with equal outcomes; however, most clinicians prefer the robust bone stock of the fibula and DCIA flap when considering dental implantology [14].

Scapular bone flaps have a low donor site morbidity and high quality of life (QOL) postoperatively making it an excellent donor site. One study looked at functional changes after a scapular tip reconstruction and found that compared to age- and sex-matched individuals, those who had scapular flaps had some decrease in shoulder strength. The average score on the simple shoulder test was 10.55 in the healthy population versus 8.31 in the study population. In orthopedic examinations, there were clinically significant differences between the controls and patients on the Patte test and external rotation lag sign test but not the external rotation test. The mean University of Washington Quality of Life was 73.39 with most patients reporting good QOL (52.6%) or very good QOL (15.7%) [15]. Overall, there were small reductions in shoulder strength and external rotation, but this did not translate into a change in QOL. There's no quality data comparing scapula tip and lateral border morbidity, but the disruption of the teres major to harvest the scapula's lateral board may cause more instability. The teres major can be preserved if only the scapular tip is harvested. When comparing QOL between the different bony donor sites, Russell et al. found no difference in global QOL score postoperatively from the baseline between fibula, scapula, and deep circumflex iliac artery reconstructions. There was a decrease in aesthetic appearance in each group postoperatively, but only fibula flap patients had significantly reduced physical activity and recreation QOL domain scores postoperatively when compared to the preoperative scores [16]. Scapula bone flaps, even when performed in a chimeric fashion with a parascapular flap, do not require skin grafting to close the donor site, unlike an osteocutaneous fibula flap. This avoids the skin graft donor site and healing of the skin graft over mobile lower extremity tendons, as with the fibula osteocutaneous flaps.

Scapular bone is an excellent donor site for bony reconstruction due to its reliable anatomy, chimeric opportunities, and low donor site morbidity. In this chapter, we will describe the indications, vascular anatomy, markings, and operative technique and present clinical cases that utilized a bony scapular flap.

Pertinent Anatomy

Blood Supply to the Lateral Scapula and Scapular Tip

The blood supply for the scapular bone flaps is based on branches of the axillary artery. As the axillary artery continues distally to the pectoralis minor, it contributes three branches before becoming the brachial artery as it passes the inferior border of the teres major. The branches are the anterior and posterior circumflex humeral arteries and the subscapular artery. Continuing distally the subscapular artery has a short course before dividing into the circumflex scapular and thoracodorsal arteries about 2–3 cm from its origin.

The circumflex scapular artery gives off a superficial branch that travels through the triangular space bordered by the teres major, teres minor, and long head of the triceps. This branch is called the superficial circumflex scapular artery and divides into the descending (vertical) and transverse (horizontal) branches to supply the parascapular and scapular fasciocutaneous flaps, respectively. The circumflex scapular artery continues inferiorly along the lateral aspect of the scapula giving off a descending branch that provides blood supply to the lateral border of the scapula and then anastomoses with branches supplied to the tip of the scapula from the angular branch of the thoracodorsal artery. The circumflex scapular artery continues to provide branches to the teres minor, teres major, and infraspinatus and then terminates as a branch to the subscapularis.

The other branch of the subscapular artery, the thoracodorsal artery, continues distally giving branches to the serratus muscle as well as a branch to the scapular tip known as the angular branch which anastomoses with the descending branch of the circumflex scapular artery (Fig. 5.1). The takeoff of the serratus and angular branches varies but anatomic studies found that 50% of the time the angular branch comes off the thoracodorsal artery distal to the branch of the serratus anterior but can come off distal or at the serratus branch [11]. The thoracodorsal artery then continues to provide the major blood supply to the latissimus dorsi muscle.

Flap Characteristics

Circumflex scapular artery: The circumflex scapular artery has a length of 5–7 cm but can be increased to 7–10 cm including the subscapular vessels from their origin. The circumflex scapular artery and venae comitantes have a size between 2.5 and 4 mm.

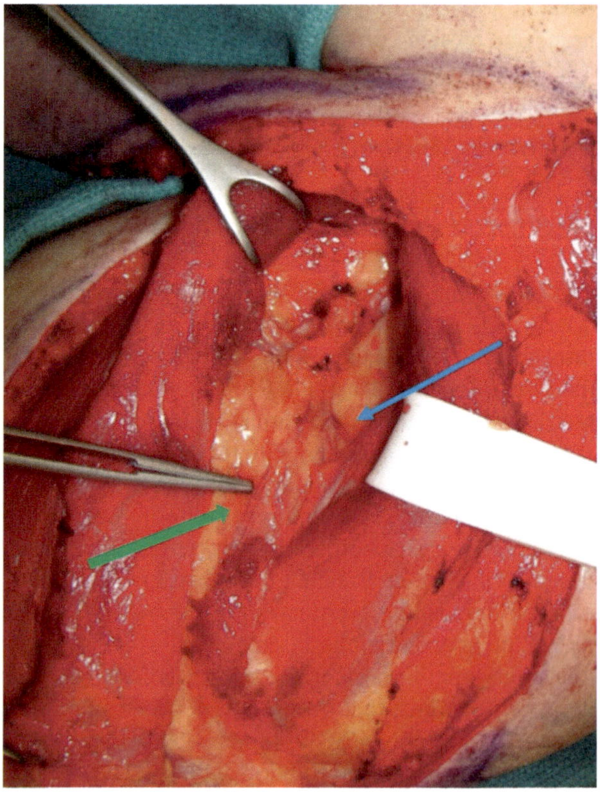

Fig. 5.1 The anatomy of the angular branch has some variations. In this dissection, the angular branch (green arrow) can be seen in the fat pad as it enters the scapula tip. The angular branch most commonly arises from the thoracodorsal artery

Angular artery: The angular artery and venae comitantes are approximately 2 mm in size and have a length between 4 and 5 cm. If dissection is carried proximal to the axillary vessels, vascularized bone supplied by the angular branch can have a pedicle length of 13–15 cm.

The distance between the bony supply point of the angular branch and the entry of the circumflex scapular artery into the bone was found to be 8–9 cm in males and 6–7 cm in females. When the circumflex scapular artery and the angular branch are connected at the subscapular artery, the two segments of the scapula can be transferred as a single bipedicled flap. These bony segments with independent blood supply can be separated by approximately 15 cm which allows for flexibility in the inset [10].

Up to 14 cm of bone can be harvested from the scapula based on the angular or circumflex scapular artery, starting 1 cm below the glenoid fossa and extending to the scapular tip [12].

Indications

The scapular flap has been described for many indications from head and neck to extremity bony reconstruction and offers advantages other bony-free flaps are unable to provide. It is commonly used in defects requiring bone as well as other tissues like the latissimus flap, which can provide a large amount of muscle, and the parascapular flap, which can provide fasciocutaneous tissue. The skin paddle of the parascapular flap can be designed up to 24 cm in length and limited to around 10 cm wide to allow for primary closure [17]. It is an excellent match for head and neck reconstruction and is usually thin and hairless. The scapular bone flap has low donor site morbidity [18, 19]. In patients with PVD, the scapular area is often spared so it is a great alternative to the fibula flap. The major disadvantage of the flap is the need for repositioning in the lateral decubitus position, although some surgeons harvest the scapula tip in a supine position [20]. Compared to the fibula, the scapula bone stock can be inadequate for osseointegrated dental implant placement.

The skin paddle of either the parascapular or scapular fasciocutaneous flap is often intermediate thickness, compared to an ALT or radial forearm flap, and should routinely be considered. In terms of aesthetic donor sites, the parascapular skin paddle harvest leaves a well-hidden scar along the posterior axillary fold and is considered superior to the scar of the scapular or horizontal skin paddle. Perhaps the only flap with a better donor site scar placement is the superficial circumflex iliac artery perforator (SCIP) flap.

Preoperative Planning

Virtual surgical planning (VSP) is used to plan the surgery in all of our free bony scapular flaps. Imaging of the scapula and axilla is obtained preoperatively and a planning session is held with the collaborative ablative and dental restoration teams when appropriate to guide the surgical planning. In maxillary reconstruction using scapular flaps, virtual surgical planning with a customized osteotomy guide has been shown to improve the quality of life in terms of pain, appearance, chewing and swallowing food, pronouncing words, and shoulder quality of life outcomes [21].

Compared to the fibula flap, the scapula has much more overlying muscular soft tissue (e.g., infraspinatus, subscapularis) so this needs to be considered when performing VSP (Fig. 5.2). The cutting guide for the scapula usually has a 5-mm offset to accommodate for soft tissues compared to 2 mm for the fibula. We also print acrylic models of the intended scapula shape and size needed in the final reconstruction for on-table fine-tuning (Fig. 5.3). There is definitely more of a learning curve to using VSP with the scapula, but with time it is a useful tool for bony reconstruction.

Markings

In the preoperative area the posterior axillary line, axillary fold, scapular lateral border, tip, and spine are marked. If designing a scapular or parascapular flap, the skin paddle must include the tissue over the triangular space, where the superficial

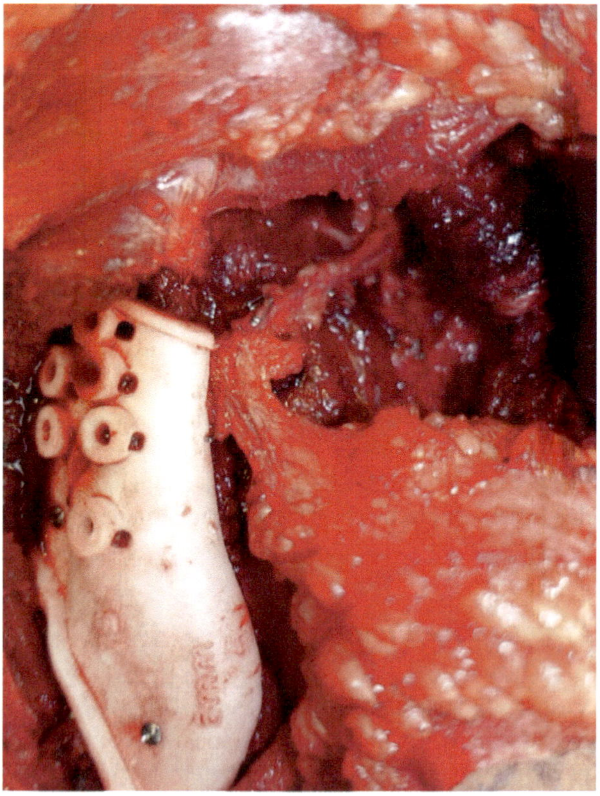

Fig. 5.2 Significant soft tissue around the scapula makes it difficult for the VSP cutting guide to be properly secured. A 5 mm offset to accommodate for soft tissues is suggested

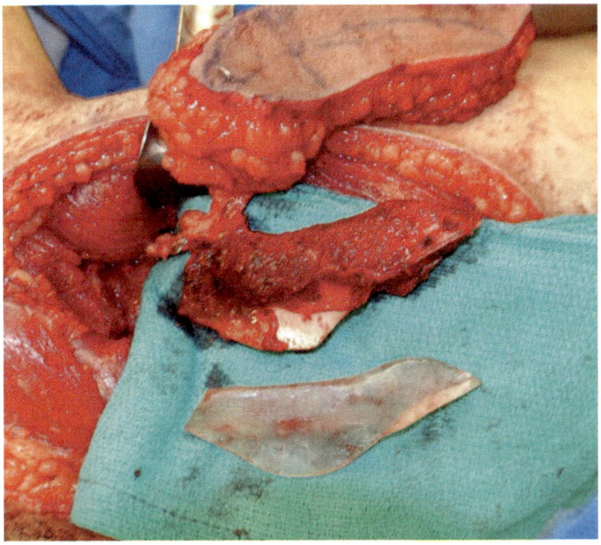

Fig. 5.3 Chimeric lateral scapula bone flap and parascapular flap in situ. Fine-tuning of the flap can be done based on the acrylic model before dividing the pedicle and transferring to the defect

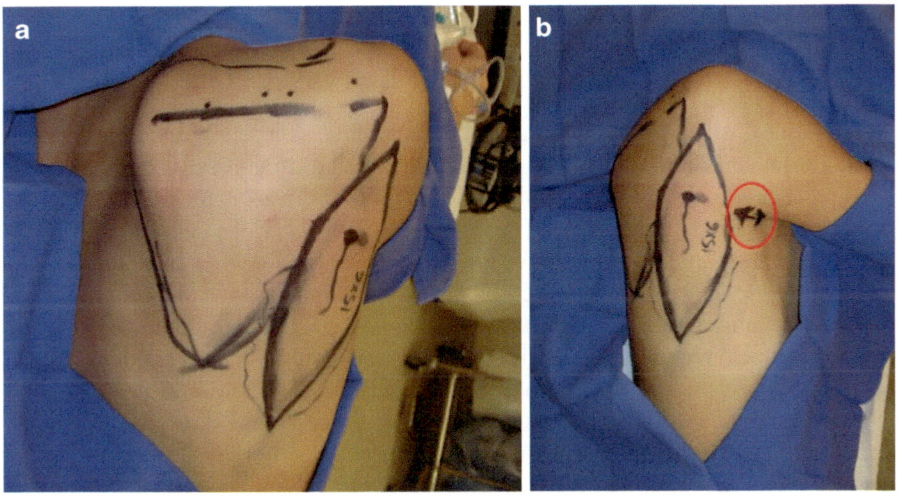

Fig. 5.4 (**a**) Markings for a bony scapula and parascapular flap are completed in the pre-operative area and confirmed once in the appropriate lateral decubitus position. The lateral border, spine, and tip of the scapula are palpated and marked. (**b**) The triangular space is marked with a dot for the anticipated location of the superficial circumflex scapular artery which is confirmed with a hand-held Doppler just where the lateral border of the scapula intersects with the continuation of the posterior axillary fold marked with a red circle

circumflex scapular artery runs through to enter the posterior fascia and the skin. The triangular space is easily palpated where the lateral border of the scapula intersects with the continuation of the posterior axillary fold (Fig. 5.4). The Doppler is used to identify the artery traveling through this space. The width of the flap is limited to allow for primary closure and skin pinch is done to mark the extent that can be harvested safely and is typically limited to 8–10 cm. Markings for the soft tissue chimeric flap must keep in mind access to the scapula.

Positioning

The patient is prepped in at least 15° of lateral to complete lateral decubitus position. The ipsilateral shoulder, back, and upper arm are circumferentially prepped to allow for mobilization of the arm and exposure of the subscapular system from an axillary approach, if necessary. To perform a bone-only scapular flap, minimal lateral decubitus position is required, but if additional flaps are being harvested, a formal lateral decubitus position may be indicated. Once the patient is positioned, the bony landmarks are again marked as the scapula position may change based on positioning. The location of the superficial circumflex scapular artery is identified using a handheld Doppler in the triangular space.

Operative Technique

As mentioned, we prefer the parascapular variant of the skin paddle and begin the dissection from caudal to cranial. Unlike an ALT flap, the circumflex scapular vessel is not a perforator and runs axially within the skin. For this reason, the vessel enters the paddle eccentrically. The flap is raised subfascially over the latissimus muscle, although some authors advocated for a suprafascial elevation. The advantage here is that the subfascial plane will more easily enable the surgeon to visualize the transition between the latissimus muscle and the teres major. These two muscles have fibers that run in the same direction so the ability to see the transition from one to another is critical (Fig. 5.5). As the surgeon approaches the caudal aspect of the teres major, the circumflex scapular vessels can be visualized within the septum that travels through the triangular space. If there is a concern about the location of the vessel, the more medial border of the skin island can be incised. In this location, you may find the transverse or scapular branch of the circumflex scapular system. This can serve as an additional reference point or clue that the surgeon is in the correct area. The teres minor can also be identified as more cephalad and has a distinctly different appearance with a more dense fascia compared to the teres major. In our experience, the triceps muscle most anteriorly does not serve as a useful clinical reference localizing the vessel.

Once the circumflex scapular vessels are identified, the triangular space can be opened more widely in the anterior direction towards the axilla. The arm should be free-draped for manipulation to open the anatomic spaces as the operation proceeds. Immediately upon entering the triangular space, there will be large branches of the circumflex scapular system that enter the lateral border of the scapula. They are tightly adherent to the bone so care must be given to avoid avulsion injury. Even when using the lateral border of the scapula in the reconstruction, usually at least the

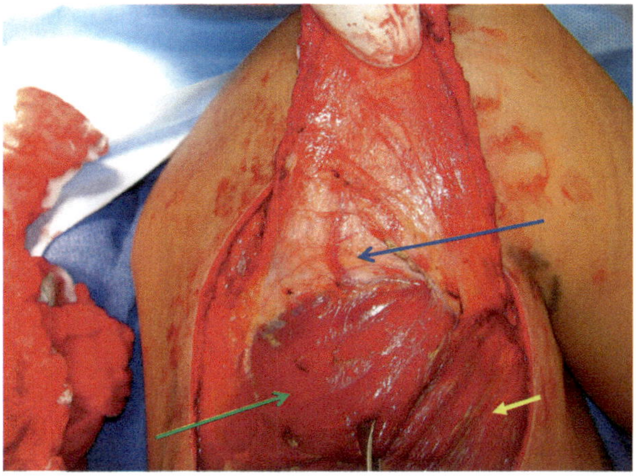

Fig. 5.5 When raising a parascapular skin paddle, the latissimus (yellow arrow) and teres major (green arrow) muscle fibers have similar orientations. When raising a fasciocutaneous parascapular flap, the blood supply is axial (blue arrow), so the flap must be raised from distal to proximal keeping the superficial circumflex scapular artery visible within the flap

most cephalad bone branch needs to be sacrificed to enable the osteotomy to be performed. For those cases in which only the soft tissue paddle is being used, this will prove to be the most difficult portion of the case.

At this point, the operation can proceed more deeply within the axilla if only a soft tissue paddle is being harvested. The surgeon can decide on the vessel length and caliber needed for the reconstruction. If significant pedicle length is needed, the thoracodorsal branch to the latissimus can be ligated without concern; however, the nerve needs to be preserved.

For cases that require a bony component, at this point, the teres major muscle is usually divided. It is ideal to divide it as close to the scapula as possible so that it can be reinserted at the end of the flap harvest (Fig. 5.6). In some cases, this muscle becomes de-vascularized and needs to be discarded. With the teres muscle reflected large bone branches can be seen entering the lateral and deep aspect of the scapula. On occasion, there are vessel branches that run on the superficial surface of the scapula. These can be preserved, but usually need to be sacrificed when making osteotomies. These are not the primary blood supply to the bone so can be safely sacrificed. If the lateral border is intended to be used in the reconstruction, the superficial muscles, such as the infraspinatus, can be removed with cautery leaving a 2–3-mm muscular cuff (Fig. 5.7a). The bone osteotomy is made proximally and distally. The final step is division of the subscapularis muscle fibers (Fig. 5.7b).

If the scapula tip is desired as a second piece of bone or as the only bony segment, then the dissection continues in the fat pad lateral to the scapula. Here the surgeon can find the thoracodorsal vessel with the angular branch emanating and joining the scapular tip. The easiest way to find the angular vessel is to retract the medial portion of the scapular tip away from the chest wall. The angular vessel will be seen as a bowstring inserting on the deep surface of the scapula. The osteotomy to the scapula tip is more straightforward than the lateral border, although the bone stock is not as robust. If additional soft tissues are needed, the latissimus muscle with or without its skin paddle can be harvested or alternatively a thoracodorsal artery perforator flap.

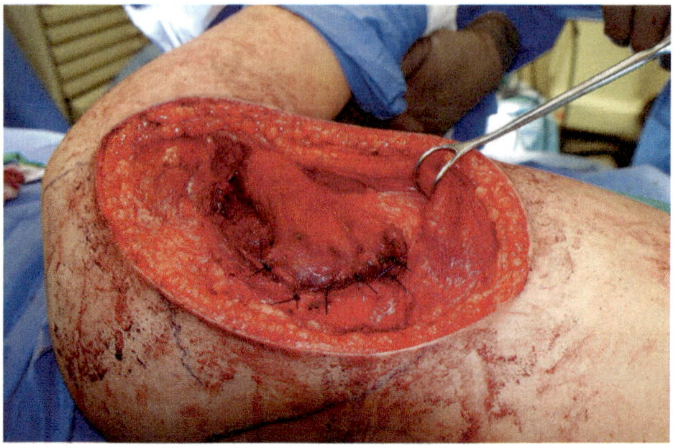

Fig. 5.6 Teres major is divided at the edge of the scapula and reinserted at the time of closure

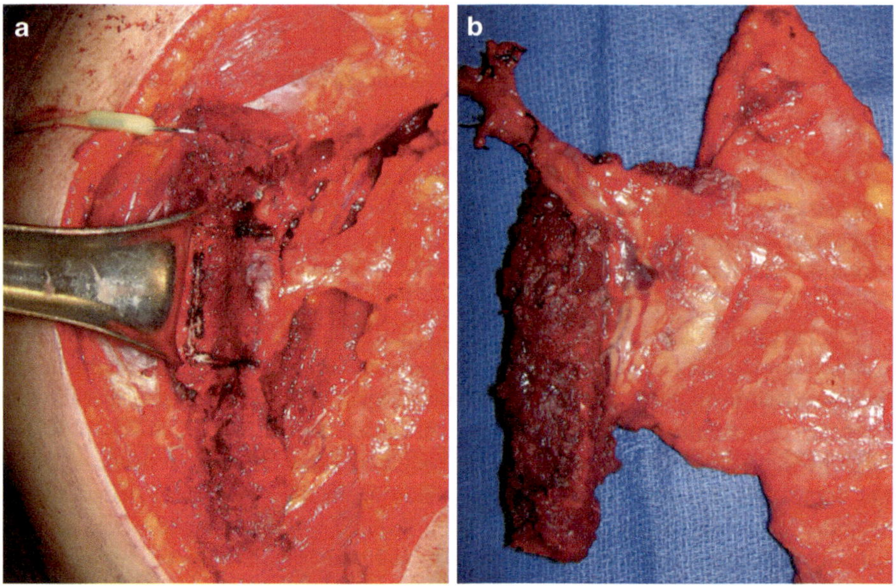

Fig. 5.7 (**a**) When harvesting the lateral scapula bone, the superficial muscles, such as the infraspinatus muscle, can be removed with cautery, leaving a 2–3 muscular cuff. This allows for sufficient exposure for a cutting guide if it is being utilized. (**b**) The final step is releasing the subscapularis muscle fibers to allow the bony segment to be mobilized from the remainder of the scapula

Clinical Cases

Case 1

The patient is a 71-year-old male with a history of type 2 diabetes mellitus, hypertension, hyperlipidemia, and significant atherosclerotic disease with a history of strokes with bilateral carotid endarterectomies and peripheral vascular disease status post bilateral lower extremity stents presenting with T4N2b stage VI squamous cell cancer of the left lower gum.

For over a year, the patient had tooth pain with loss of intermittent teeth requiring some narcotic medication and was trialed on antibiotics with no resolution of his symptoms. The patient had 18 teeth removed by his dentist and the left lower gum failed to heal. A biopsy of the nonhealing ulcer in the left lower anterior gum showed squamous cell cancer, moderately differentiated.

On exam, the oral cavity showed an exophytic tumor filling the anterior mandible and left body of the mandible that extended across to the right canine tooth. Palpation showed infiltration into the gingivobuccal sulcus anteriorly and gingivolabial sulcus and external mental skin changes. Imaging demonstrated a 5.1-cm mass in length from the symphysis to the left angle in addition to a left level 1B necrotic node, 1.15 cm in size (Fig. 5.8). The patient underwent neoadjuvant chemotherapy with an overall decrease in the size of the soft tissue mass along the left anterior gingivobuccal sulcus. He had a full cardiac workup and was cleared for surgery.

Preoperative imaging was obtained of his bilateral lower extremities and a CT angiogram demonstrated significant atherosclerotic disease with calcifications throughout his vessels. The dominant vessel single runoff to the foot appears to be the peroneal artery (Fig. 5.9). Given the findings on his CT angiogram, the decision was made to proceed with a chimeric right scapular flap with a parascapular skin island and possible latissimus flap. Given his comorbidities, he would be a poor candidate for simultaneous two-free-flap reconstruction. VSP was used to perform the planning of the resection and two-segment scapular flap (Fig. 5.10).

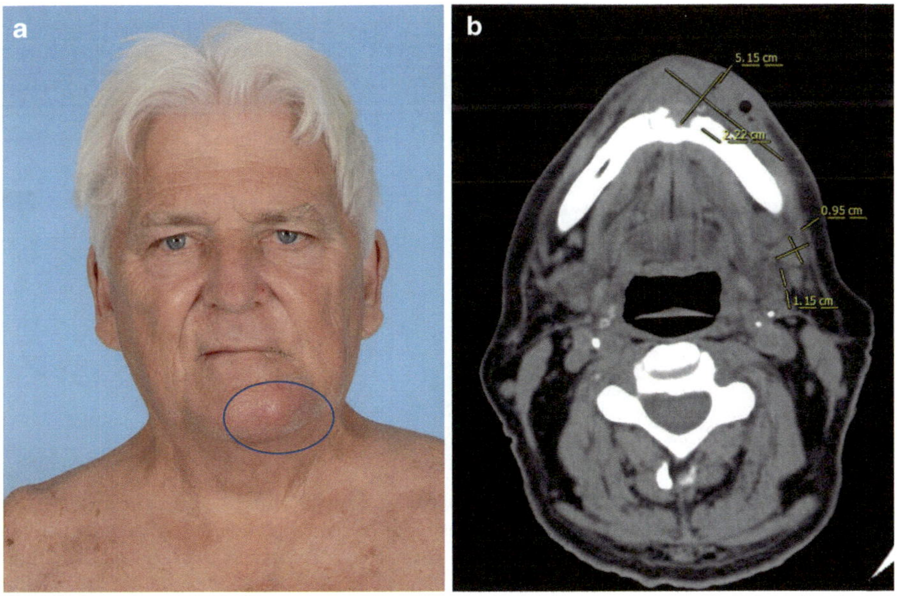

Fig. 5.8 (**a**) Pre-operative photograph with skin changes to the left mental region. (**b**) CT axial cross section with large erosive tumor with associated necrotic level 1B lymph node

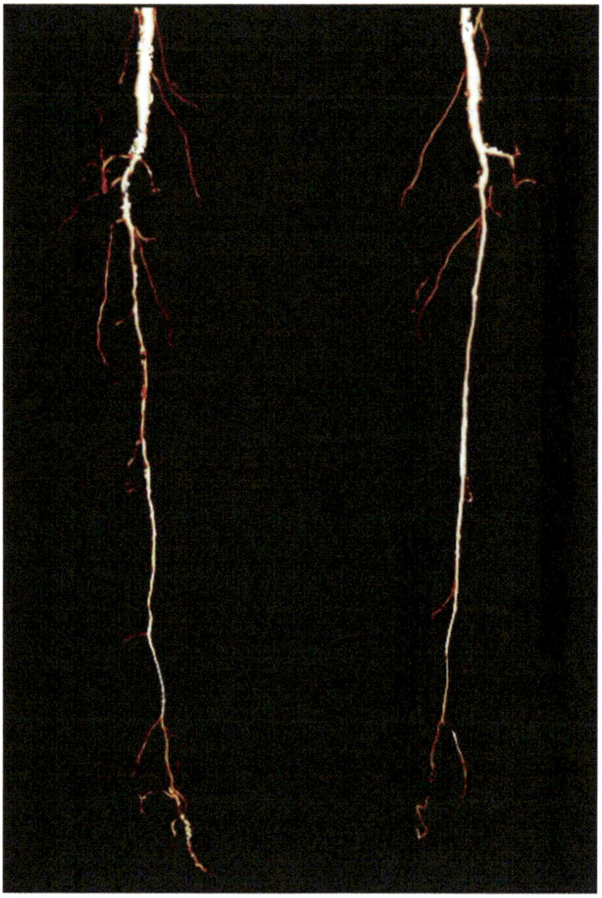

Fig. 5.9 CT angiogram of bilateral lower extremities demonstrating severe peripheral vascular disease with the peroneal vessel as the one vessel runoff to the feet eliminating a free fibula flap for reconstruction of the mandibular defect

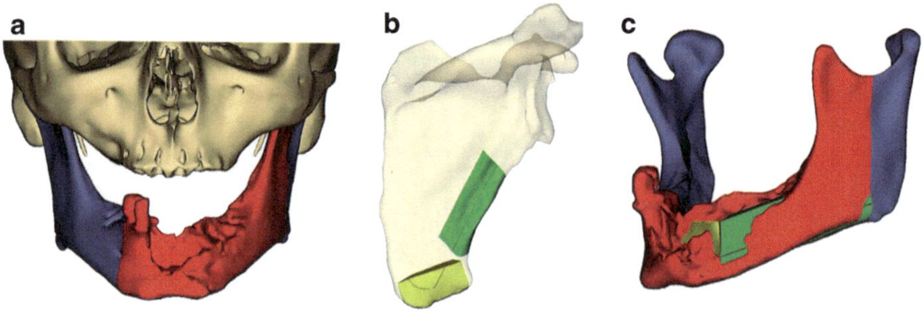

Fig. 5.10 (**a**) VSP planning highlighting osteotomy sites with red being the resected mandible. (**b**) VSP planning of the scapular two-bone segments with the green portion delineating the body of the scapula supplied by the descending branch of the circumflex scapular artery and the yellow portion of the tip of the scapula supplied by the angular branch. (**c**) VSP overlay of the planned resection in red and the two-bone scapular segments in yellow and green

In a combined approach with the head and neck service, the patient underwent a mandibulectomy from the right parasymphysis to the trans-mandibular notch and resection of a portion of that anterior floor of the mouth and mental skin, left 1–4 node dissection, and tracheostomy. The reconstruction consisted of a two-segment bone flap from the scapula based on the circumflex scapular and angular arteries and two skin paddles, parascapular and myocutaneous latissimus. The bony segments were plated in situ before transfer to the recipient site (Fig. 5.11). The construct was then plated to the native mandible and the intraoral parascapular skin paddle was inset (Fig. 5.12). The microvascular anastomosis was then completed followed by reconstruction of the external chin defect with myocutaneous latissimus skin paddle.

Overall, the patient did well postoperatively. There was no detectable tumor in the specimen after this induction chemotherapy. There were no flap complications and he progressed well. He had a PEG tube placed to maximize nutrition by the interventional radiology team and was discharged home on post-op day 14. The

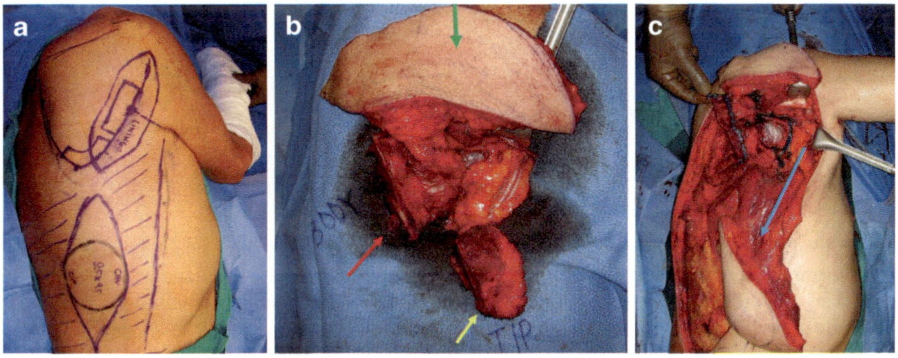

Fig. 5.11 (**a**) Markings for chimeric two-segment bone scapular flap, parascapular flap, and myocutaneous latissimus flap. (**b**) Green arrow—parascapular flap, red arrow—body of scapula, yellow arrow—tip of scapula. (**c**) Plating of the two-bone segments in situ and myocutaneous latisimuss flap (blue arrow)

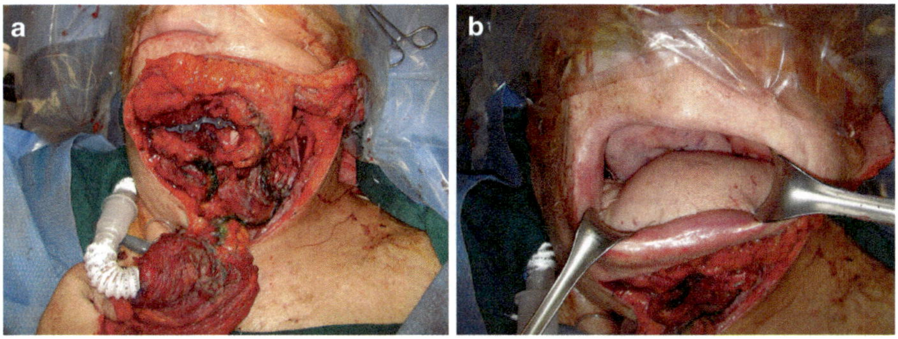

Fig. 5.12 (**a**) Two-segment bone scapular flap fixated to the native remaining mandible. (**b**) Intraoral inset of parascapular flap

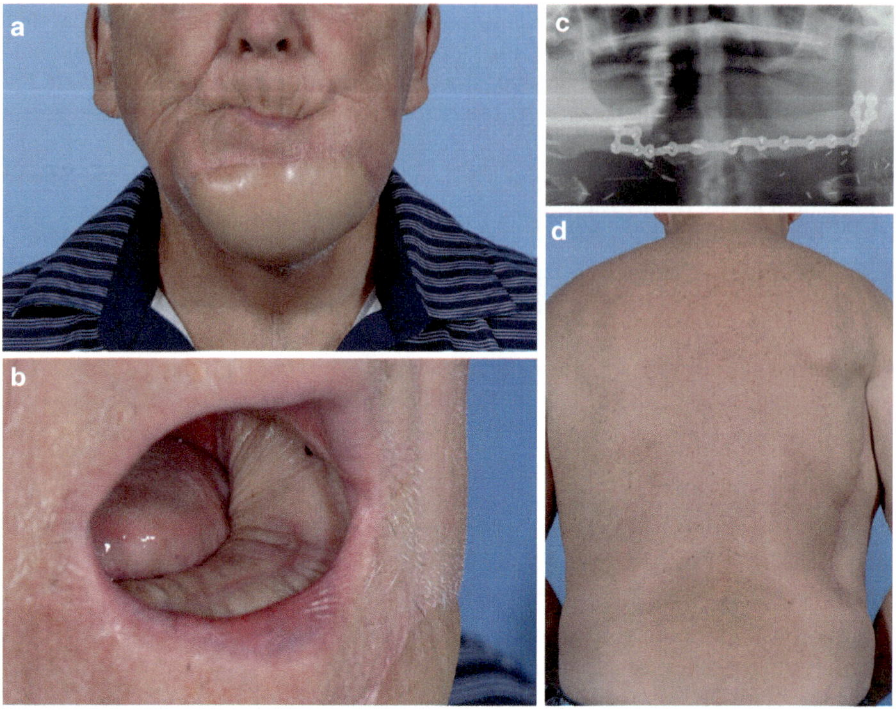

Fig. 5.13 (**a**) Post-operative extraoral myocutaneous latissimus flap after one debulking. Patient demonstrating adequate oral competence. (**b**) Well-healed intraoral parascapular flap after one debulking procedure. (**c**) Panorex of mandibular fixation. (**d**) Extended longitudinal scar from chimeric scapular flap including latissimus muscle

patient did have pain in the right shoulder and limited range of motion and was seen by the orthopedic team. The workup found arthritis in his right shoulder and the pain was relieved with a corticosteroid injection. Four months after surgery the patient returned to the operating room for debulking and contouring of the intraoral parascapular and extraoral myocutaneous latissimus flaps with a combination of liposuction and direct excision which resulted in a satisfactory aesthetic outcome and adequate oral competence. His hardware was confirmed to be in good position on imaging (Fig. 5.13). He has had his PEG tube removed and has returned to his preoperative diet and activity.

Case 2

The patient is a 17-year-old male diagnosed with a high-grade osteosarcoma of the right femur at age 11. He was treated with induction chemotherapy followed by a femur resection complicated by infection and revision of the knee prosthetic. He developed metastasis to the lungs and underwent wedge resection and chemotherapy. He now presents with new-onset jaw pain.

The patient's symptoms initially started with some chin and lip numbness on the left with subsequent pain and discomfort. Imaging demonstrated a lesion within the ramus of the mandible, 2.6 x 2.1 cm in size with extraosseous extension, and with infiltration of the pterygoid muscle, masseter muscle, and the mandible foramen and inferior alveolar canal (Fig. 5.14). A biopsy confirmed the mass as metastatic osteosarcoma, and he was started on neoadjuvant chemotherapy.

On exam there were noted to be changes to the mucosa intraorally, but no erosive changes to the mucosa with intact facial nerve function. He has mild to moderate soft tissues over the scapula. He has had a left thoracotomy. He has moderate soft tissue thickness over his thighs and the fibula donor site.

In counseling for this patient's reconstruction soft tissue only and a combination of bony and soft tissue reconstruction were discussed. The benefits of bony reconstruction include improved facial contour and avoiding malocclusion by maintaining a posterior height on the left side of the neoramus construct. The potential of a chimeric scapular flap and a left osteocutaneous fibula flap were both options in his case, but given his prior lower extremity surgeries the plan was to avoid extensive dissection of the lower extremity when only a small segment of bone would need to be harvested. For this reason, the scapula was chosen as the donor site. VSP was used to determine the resection and the scapular bone flap (Fig. 5.15).

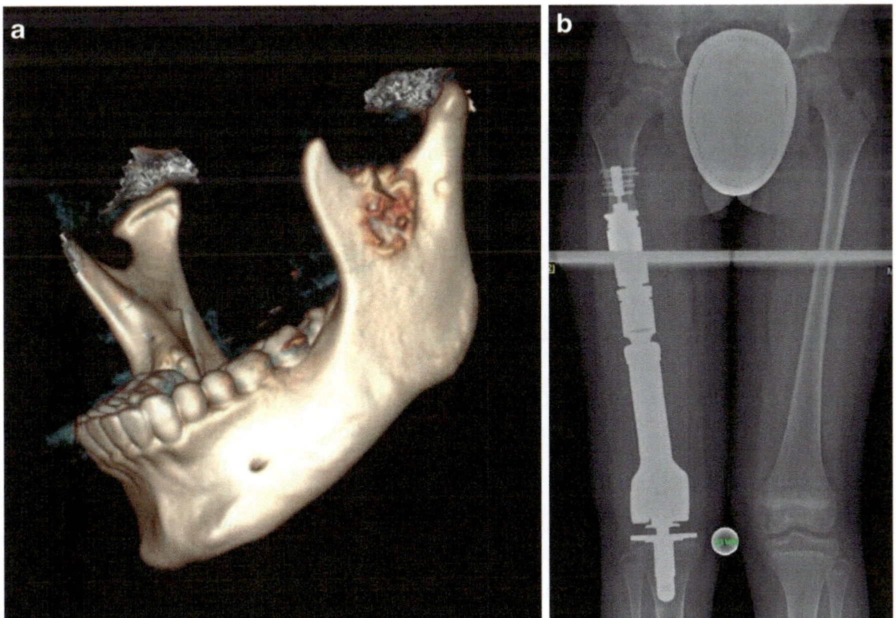

Fig. 5.14 (**a**) CT 3D reconstruction of lesion within the ramus of the mandible, 2.6 × 2.1 cm in size with extraosseous extension. (**b**) Imaging of bilateral lower extremities with prosthesis in the right femur and knee from prior osteosarcoma resection

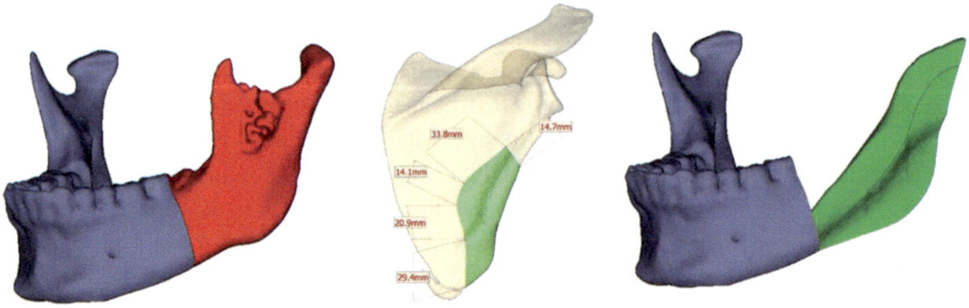

Fig. 5.15 VSP planning of resection in red. Planned single segment scapular bone flap in green

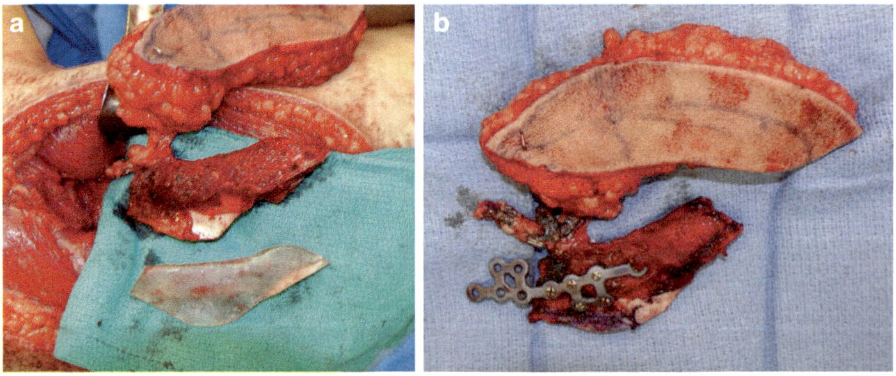

Fig. 5.16 (**a**) Chimeric variant with scapular bone segment and parascapular flap based on circumflex scapular artery. Bony model used for fine tuning. (**b**) Chimeric flap with hardware that had been fixated to scapular bone segment before dividing the pedicle

In combination with the head and neck service the patient underwent composite resection of the mandible ramus and posterior body en bloc, with contents of left masticator space and infratemporal fossa and left neck dissection levels 1B and 2A. The reconstruction included the left hemimandible defect with a chimeric parascapular and scapular bone flap. The flap included one bony segment and was fixated in situ before transecting the pedicle and transferring to the defect (Fig. 5.16). The parascapular flap was inset to the posterior intraoral defect, followed by fixation to the native mandible, and microsurgical anastomosis (Fig. 5.17).

The patient progressed well after surgery. He was started on an oral diet on postoperative day 10 and was discharged home on postoperative day 13. The patient was continued on chemotherapy and immunotherapy and unfortunately has developed other sites of metastatic disease. His intraoral flap healed well with good contour and bony reconstruction with stable fixation on imaging. His right donor site healed well without donor site morbidity (Fig. 5.18).

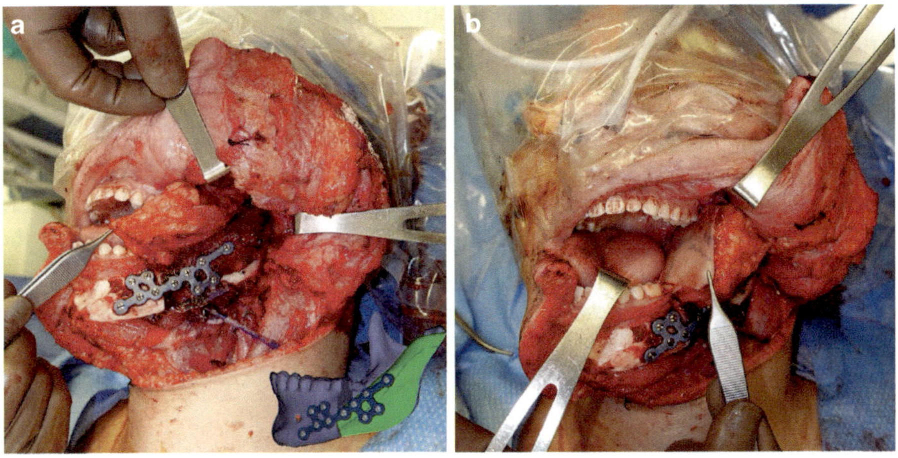

Fig. 5.17 (**a**) Rigid fixation of the scapular flap to the native mandible. (**b**) Inset of parascapular flap into the intraoral defect

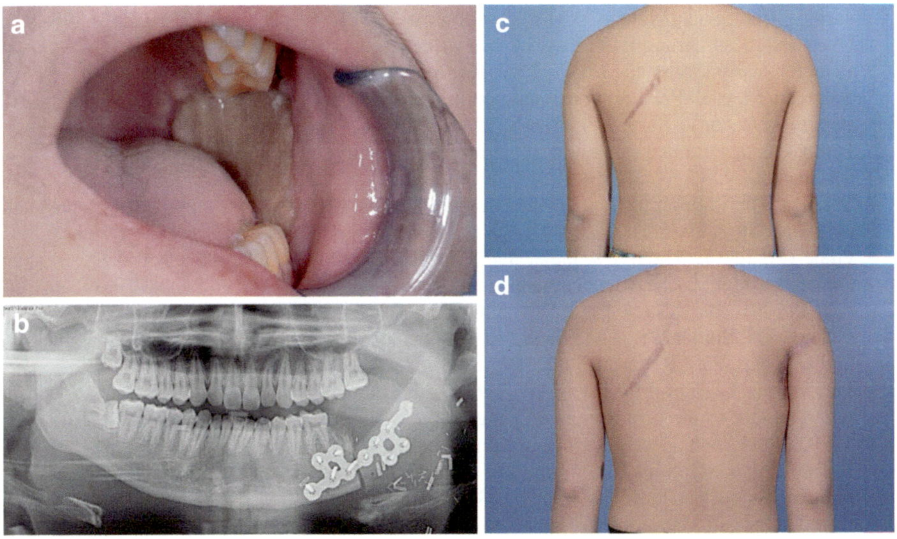

Fig. 5.18 (**a**) Well-healed intraoral parascapular flap with good contour. (**b**) Early stable fixation on post-operative panorex. (**c**) Pre-operative photograph with thoracotomy incision on the left. (**d**) Post-operative photograph with a well-concealed and healed scar on the right from parascapular and scapular bone flap

Summary

Scapular bone has been well established as a safe reliable donor site for vascularized bone flaps with minimal and acceptable donor site morbidity. A wide array of defects have been reconstructed with scapular bone. The anatomy is consistent with two segments of bone that can be utilized based on the circumflex scapular artery or the angular artery to harvest the lateral scapula and scapular tip. Additional tissue including muscle, fascia, and skin can be harvested to create chimeric flaps based on the subscapular system. VSP can be utilized to perform presurgical planning. Scapular bone flaps should be considered in complex cases that require multiple tissue types and/or when the fibula flap is contraindicated. The parascapular fasciocutaneous flap is an excellent donor site with a relatively inconspicuous scar so should be routinely considered as an alternative to the ALT flap.

References

1. Patel SY, Kim DD, Ghali GE. Maxillofacial reconstruction using vascularized fibula free flaps and endosseous implants. Oral Maxillofac Surg Clin North Am. 2019;31(2):259–84.
2. Shahzad F, et al. Reconstruction of oncologic upper extremity defects with fibula free flaps has high union rates and excellent functional outcomes. J Surg Oncol. 2023;128(8):1416–27.
3. Weichman KE, et al. Lower extremity osseous oncologic reconstruction with composite microsurgical free fibula inside massive bony allograft. Plast Reconstr Surg. 2015;136(2):396–403.
4. Riasa INP, Kawilarang B. The use of free vascularized fibula graft in spinal reconstruction: a comprehensive systematic review. Plast Reconstr Surg Glob Open. 2023;11(6):e5079.
5. Sakuraba M, et al. Pelvic ring reconstruction with the double-barreled vascularized fibular free flap. Plast Reconstr Surg. 2005;116(5):1340–5.
6. Hallock GG. Permutations of combined free flaps using the subscapular system. J Reconstr Microsurg. 1997;13(1):47–54.
7. Saijo M. The vascular territories of the dorsal trunk: a reappraisal for potential flap donor sites. Br J Plast Surg. 1978;31(3):200–4.
8. Gilbert A, Teot L. The free scapular flap. Plast Reconstr Surg. 1982;69(4):601–4.
9. Swartz WM, et al. The osteocutaneous scapular flap for mandibular and maxillary reconstruction. Plast Reconstr Surg. 1986;77(4):530–45.
10. Coleman JJ, Sultan MR. The bipedicled osteocutaneous scapula flap: a new subscapular system free flap. Plast Reconstr Surg. 1991;87(4):682–92.
11. Seneviratne S, Duong C, Taylor GI. The angular branch of the thoracodorsal artery and its blood supply to the inferior angle of the scapula: an anatomical study. Plast Reconstr Surg. 1999;104(1):85–8.
12. Hasan Z, et al. Options for configuring the scapular free flap in maxillary, mandibular, and calvarial reconstruction. Plast Reconstr Surg. 2013;132(3):645–55.
13. Harada H, et al. Mandibular reconstruction with scapular systems: a single-center case series involving 208 flaps. Plast Reconstr Surg. 2021;148(3):625–34.
14. Wilkman T, Husso A, Lassus P. Clinical comparison of scapular, fibular, and iliac crest osseal free flaps in maxillofacial reconstructions. Scand J Surg. 2019;108(1):76–82.
15. Valentini V, et al. The use of scapular bone flaps during head-and-neck reconstruction: functional, orthopedic, and quality of life analyses of flap-harvest-related deficits. J Craniofac Surg. 2022;33(7):2031–4.
16. Russell J, et al. Implications of the composite free flap harvest site on quality of life after head and neck surgery: a prospective series. Int J Oral Maxillofac Surg. 2024;53(4):275–81.
17. Hamilton SG, Morrison WA. The scapular free flap. Br J Plast Surg. 1982;35(1):2–7.
18. Ranganath K, et al. Comparison of patient-reported upper extremity disability following free flaps in head and neck reconstruction: a systematic review and meta-analysis. Head Neck. 2023;45(7):1832–40.

19. Ferrari S, et al. Donor site morbidity after scapular tip free flaps in head-and-neck reconstruction. Microsurgery. 2015;35(6):447–50.
20. Miyamoto S, et al. Scapula harvest in the supine position for immediate mandibular reconstruction. Oral Maxillofac Surg. 2024;28:1181.
21. Alwadeai M, et al. Virtual surgical guidance improves quality of life following scapular free-flap reconstruction of maxillary defects. J Oral Maxillofac Surg. 2024;82:600.

Chapter 6
Great Toe and Second Toe Transfer

Steven J. Lo, Jennifer Ling, and Fu Chan Wei

History

In 1898 Nicoladoni performed the world's first pedicled toe-to-hand transplantation. This represented a paradigm shift from his earlier attempts at thumb reconstruction with tubed chest flaps, which could not achieve a like-for-like reconstruction of a thumb [21]. However, this did not result in the expected revolution in hand reconstruction, perhaps as patients still had to endure months with the hand attached to the foot, with only a few sporadic reports in the ensuing decades [4]. It was not until the advent of microsurgery, which permitted single stage toe-to-hand transfer, when toe transfer finally revolutionized the field of hand surgery. This began initially with the experimental work of Buncke in 1964 in a Rhesus monkey [2], followed shortly thereafter by Yang from China and Cobbett from the United Kingdom [1, 5]. A period of intense innovation arose in the 1980s with the description of the trimmed toe, twisted toe, vascularised joint transfer, toe pulp and wraparound flaps [9, 27, 31].

Research has indicated the superiority of free toe transplantation over revision amputation or conventional methods such as osteoplastic reconstruction,

S. J. Lo
Canniesburn Plastic Surgery Unit, Glasgow Royal Infirmary, Glasgow, UK

School of Medicine, Dentistry & Nursing, University of Glasgow, Glasgow, UK

J. Ling
Department of Plastic and Reconstructive Surgery, Chang Gung Memorial Hospital, Taoyuan, Taiwan

F. C. Wei (✉)
Department of Plastic and Reconstructive Surgery, Chang Gung Memorial Hospital, Taoyuan, Taiwan

Chang Gung University, Medical College, Taoyuan, Taiwan

J. P. Agarwal, D. W. Mathes (eds.), *Bone Flaps in Reconstructive Surgery*,
https://doi.org/10.1007/978-3-032-12540-8_6

particularly for thumb reconstruction [3]. However, toe-to-finger transfer is more debatable, particularly regarding single finger and partial finger loss [7]. Current data on functional recovery in toe transfers indicates sensory recovery of static 2 point discrimination of 10–11 mm in a systematic review of 450 toe to thumb transfers, with no difference noted between second toe, great toe, wrap-around or trimmed toe techniques [17]. Children show improved sensory recovery than in adults, with large series in congenital anomalies noting a static 2PD of approximately 5 mm [8, 15, 22]. In adults active ROM is about 45% of normal, with toe to thumb transfers total active ROM 65–110° and toe to finger transfers 110° [16, 17]. This impacts on the ability of toe transfers to make an effective ulnar hook or power grip, which we discuss later. Additionally, second toe transfers are weaker than great toe transfers with power grip strength after great toe to thumb transfer 78–86% of the contralateral hand, whereas in second toe transfer to thumb grip strength is 69% of the contralateral hand [17].

Our work in Chang Gung Memorial Hospital now centres around providing validated evidence from patient-reported outcomes to support long-term functional efficacy of toe transfers and also evaluation of the donor site deficits (or lack thereof) in the foot [19, 25]. Early evaluation of data from a large series with long-term follow-up of 22 years suggests that toe transfers outperform equivalent finger replantations when evaluated with the Michigan Hand Questionnaire.

In this chapter we discuss indications for great toe and second toe transfers and the pertinent anatomy and surgical approach, supported by relevant case examples.

Indications

Careful patient selection is central to a successful toe transfer outcome. Although we can provide general indications, the reconstructive plan should be tailored for each patient rather than simply based on the injury phenotype. For example, patient wishes, occupation, functional and psychological needs and cultural expectations should be factored into the decision-making process. The congenital hand is a separate topic in its own right, although toe transfers play a crucial role in the reconstruction of defects such as symbrachydactyly, constriction ring and thumb hypoplasia and have been described in large series worldwide [8, 14, 22].

Thumb Reconstruction

Loss of the thumb is one of the strongest indications for toe transfer. Thumb function decreases by 50% with amputations at the level of the interphalangeal joint (IPJ) and reaches 100% proximal to the metacarpophalangeal joint (MCPJ) [24]. Although there are numerous approaches to great toe transfer in isolated thumb amputations, our preferred approach is the trimmed great toe, first described by Wei in 1983. The trimmed toe approach allows a one-stage volume reduction technique that allows a better aesthetic match between the great toe and thumb. It has significant advantages over other volume reduction techniques such as the wraparound technique, which has significant donor site morbidity, lack of interphalangeal joint (IPJ) mobility and iliac bone-related issues of fracture and resorption. In a series of 26 trimmed great toe cases in 1988, an IPJ ROM of 18° was noted, which is slightly less than for whole great toe at 33°, but with a significantly improved neo-thumb appearance [17, 26].

The strength of indications for toe transfer to thumb differ according to amputation level. For amputations distal to the IPJ this is only a relative indication. Certain patients may benefit from fine dexterity (e.g. artists, musicians) although del Pinal has noted that manual workers also derive significant benefits [7]. For amputations *proximal to the IPJ* this is a strong indication from a functional standpoint [3], whilst those *proximal to the MCPJ* are also a strong indication, but will need to consider bone lengthening with iliac bone or distraction osteogenesis prior to toe transfer [12].

Finger Reconstruction

The indications for finger reconstruction are less well established, and it is important to note that each digit does not contribute equally to hand function and provides support to specific prehension patterns. The functional side of the digits—that is the radial pulp of the index and middle finger and the ulnar side of the thumb—are more important for digital manipulation and dexterity [31]. In multiple-digit amputations, reconstruction of a three-digit hand to enable tripod pinch and thereby functional opposition is critical. This is supported by our recent data indicating that tripod grip strength is one of the key factors that strongly influences patient-reported functional outcomes, as measured with the Michigan Hand Questionnaire [19]. Although a preference has been expressed for reconstructing the ulnar digits (middle and little fingers), particularly in the congenital hand, to provide for powerful power grip and span grips, this may not be possible due to the limited range of motion of toe transfers [14, 22, 27, 31]. Our approach is therefore to preferentially reconstruct the radial digits (index and middle, or middle and ring) to enable restoration of the tripod pinch, rather than focusing on power grip.

In single-digit reconstructions the second toe transfer is preferred. Our preference for multidigit adjacent amputations that are proximal to the webspaces is the combined second and third toe transfer, which we described in 25 cases in our early series in 1989 [29], although we have now performed over 200. For non-adjacent amputations, or those adjacent amputations distal to the webspaces, we employ bilateral second toe transfers which we have previously described in 140 cases with 98.9% survival rate [6]. This avoids the 'pseudo-syndactyly' appearance if a combined second and third toe were used.

For finger reconstruction the indications for toe transfer again vary according to amputation level and number of digits. *For single digit distal to PIPJ* this is only a relative indication [7]. *Single digit proximal to PIPJ* is seldom an indication for toe transfer, and one should be very selective due to the short length of the toe, which would result in a non-uniform finger cascade. *Multiple digits amputated distal to the webspaces* are a strong indication for bilateral second toe transfers. *Multiple digits proximal to the webspaces* are also a strong indication, but our preference here is for combined second and third toe transfers that include the toe webspace. *Multiple digits including the thumb* are a strong indication for toe transfer, with the goal of a three-digit reconstruction to enable tripod pinch. A staged approach is preferred, when the thenar muscles or basal joint is not functioning well, with reconstruction of the opposing fingers performed prior to thumb reconstruction. This allows the intervening use of a prosthetic thumb to calculate the desired rotation angle and length for neo-thumb inset, prior to toe to thumb transfer. *Metacarpal-like and metacarpal hand amputations* are strong indications for toe transfer, but the discussion of these types of injuries is outside the scope of this chapter.

Consideration of the Donor Feet

Our recent data shows no difference in patient-reported outcomes of toe transfer feet (after trimmed great toe transfer) compared to controls, using the validated Foot Function Index [25]. However, it should be noted that the technique evaluated in this study preserved the proximal 1 cm of the proximal phalanx, thereby partially maintaining the windlass mechanism of the medial plantar arch. Donor site cosmesis, particularly in the paediatric or young female patients, should be considered in deciding the appropriate toes to harvest and it is for this reason that the majority of congenital hand surgeons will use the second toe in preference to the great toe [14, 22]. Athletes and others with higher demands on foot function may also express a preference for alternative forms of hand reconstruction.

Anatomy and Dissection Technique

Anatomy

Historically, one of the most pertinent aspects of toe transfer anatomy was the different pedicle arterial systems of the first metatarsal artery system, discussed and classified by Gilbert in 1976 [11]. In this description, based on injection studies of 50 cadaveric feet, the first dorsal metatarsal artery (FDMA) was dominant in 80% of cases, and the first plantar metatarsal artery (FPMA) dominant in 20%. Although multiple classifications exist, these have now been rendered relatively obsolete due to a change in surgical approach from an antegrade technique to a retrograde first

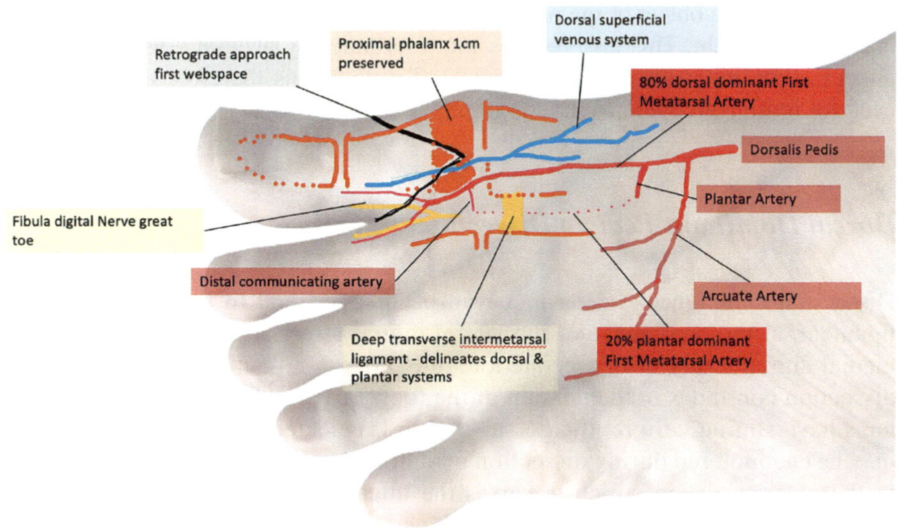

Fig. 6.1 Relevant anatomy for great toe or second toe dissection

webspace approach [11, 20, 34]. Additionally, this makes knowledge regarding absence of the dorsalis pedis in 6% [23] or the arcuate system in 40% [10] less important (Fig. 6.1).

Dissection Technique

Design of Incisions

The approach for the great toe transfer and second toe transfer is similar, although the design of the incision lines for every type of toe flap differs. Dorsal and plantar 'V-shaped' flaps are designed to facilitate inset into the 'cruciate' incision (resulting in four equal flaps) in the amputation stump. Incisions are placed off the weight-bearing plantar surfaces and an extensile dorsal lazy 'S' incision is used for exposure of a dorsal dominant system.

Retrograde Dissection of the Vascular Pedicle

Previously, most surgical techniques commenced with a vascular dissection proximally at the dorsalis pedis artery and until its continuity or lack thereof with the FDMA. However, it is easier to perform dissection in the first webspace in a retrograde manner [32], which enables the dominant vascular supply of the toe to be established at the outset of the procedure, eliminating unnecessary dissection of an inadequate pedicle. This also reduces foot morbidity by avoiding dissection of an unnecessarily long dorsalis pedis pedicle. Together, this therefore eliminates the need for routine preoperative arteriography of the foot.

Dorsal Dominant Pedicle Dissection

Dissection commences in the first webspace superficial to the intermetatarsal ligament, at the confluence of the lateral digital artery of the great toe and the medial digital artery of the second toe. In FDMA dominant systems, retrograde dissection continues in the dorsum of the foot. In 10% of cases, when both systems have similar calibre, the dorsal system is selected. A number of branches may be encountered during dissection including the distal communicating artery to the plantar system which traverses the interosseus muscle perpendicularly, the plantar artery which is the communicating branch at the base of the first metatarsal and the arcuate artery (equivalent to the dorsal arch) at the medial cuneiform. The FDMA is isolated proximally until the desired pedicle length is obtained, with intramuscular dissection where required. The FDMA tends to be apposed on the first metatarsal bone rather than the midline of the interosseus muscle; therefore, dissection should be preferentially started towards the first metatarsal [13]. Excess fatty tissues around the nerves and vessels are meticulously removed.

Plantar Dominant Pedicle Dissection

Again, a plantar dominant FPMA is recognized early with a retrograde dissection technique. An extension of the plantar skin incision should be made, lateral to the first metatarsal head to avoid scar on weight-bearing areas. The dissection does not extend beyond the middle metatarsal shaft, to reduce foot morbidity, and a vein graft is used if additional pedicle length is required.

Skeletonization of Vessels and Nerves

Our preference is to strip off the surrounding tissues from the vessels to minimize postoperative vasospasm. This not only provides mechanical release from constriction but also results in a distal sympathectomy, making vessels less prone to sympathetic influence. A skeletonized vessel also enables easier inset of the toe transfer in the hand, minimizing bulk in subcutaneous tunnels and thereby vascular compression.

Partial Preservation of the Proximal Phalanx of the Great Toe

For great toe harvest, at least 1.0 cm of the proximal phalanx is preserved. This maintains effective push-off of the donor foot associated with the windlass mechanism of the medial plantar arch, as demonstrated in plantar pressure profile studies [25]. Disarticulation through the first metatarsophalangeal joint should thus be avoided. If additional length is required for a great toe transfer, for example, in proximal thumb amputations at the metacarpal base, a first-stage iliac bone transfer with pedicled groin flap should be performed.

Skeletal and Tendon Dissection

When a metatarsal osteotomy is required to lengthen a second toe transfer, the resultant metatarsal space does not require approximation by wiring or bone blocks. No improvement has been found in gait analysis following the use of these techniques, and we therefore no longer recommend these approaches [30]. Extensor hallucis longus is taken for great toe extension and flexor hallucis ongus for flexion. Extensor hallucis brevis and extensor digitorum brevis are generally not used for reconstruction except in unusual circumstances (e.g. EDB abductoroplasty with second toe transfers for proximal thumb reconstruction). More recently, we have introduced toe transfer intrinsic reconstruction to provide a degree of dynamic reduction of extensor lag. This uses flexor digitorum sublimis tendon to intrinsic toe transfer to improve extensor lag when the fingers are flexed at the metacarpophalangeal joint [18].

Inset

The details of inset, toe transfer design in multidigit and metacarpal hand amputations, rehabilitation and post-operative management are outside the scope of this chapter and have been described extensively elsewhere [12, 27, 30].

Case Examples

Case 1: Trimmed Great Toe

The whole great toe is 80% larger in volume than the thumb, and the trimmed toe was developed by Wei in 1983 with aesthetic volume reduction in mind [26]. It remains the first choice reconstruction at Chang Gung Memorial Hospital for isolated thumb amputation. Nonetheless, patients must accept potential minor functional loss associated with reduced IP joint mobility—which may be of more importance in heavy manual labourers. Here we illustrate the case of a trimmed great toe in a 22-year-old male patient who suffered an amputation of the left non-dominant thumb through the base of the proximal phalanx in 1996 (Fig. 6.2a).

The thumb circumference of the contralateral thumb was measured at the eponychium, IP joint and mid-proximal phalanx and transposed to the great toe. A medial skin flap was marked on the great toe and measured about 12 mm in width (Fig. 6.2b and c) with care taken to preserve the paronychial fold of the great toenail. The medial skin flap was raised initially only down to just superficial to the medial collateral ligament. The second incision then was made all the way down to the bone, this layer consisting of the collateral ligament joint capsule and periosteum was raised as a 'peri-joint' flap until the middle of the plantar surface of the great toe. A longitudinal resection of a 3–5 mm width of the medial side of the joint was performed with oscillating saw, permitting osseus volume reduction, and the excess of the peri-joint flap was trimmed to allow tight closure of the joint. The medial great toe incision was closed directly prior to transfer to the hand (Fig. 6.2d).

At 1-year follow-up the aesthetic and functional results were excellent. Note that the patient had already undergone pulp-plasty to further reduce pulp volume (Fig. 6.2e and f). This is safe to perform 3 months post-operatively, and in our series of 82 patients scar hypersensitivity was not found to be an issue [33]. At 20-year

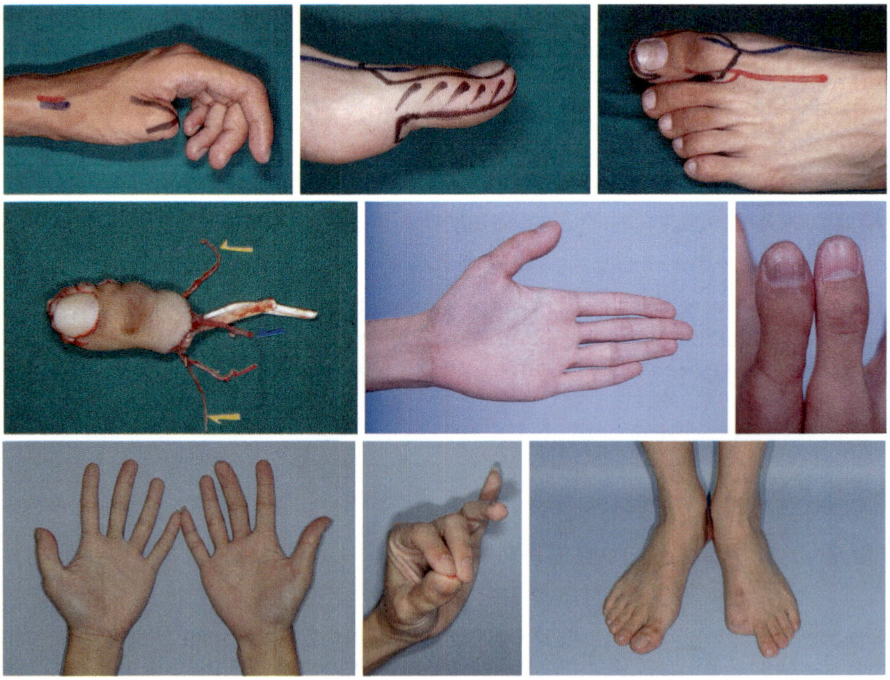

Fig. 6.2 Trimmed great toe sequence of surgical steps

follow-up in 2016, the aesthetic and functional results remained stable and the patient was delighted with the long-term results (Fig. 6.2g and h). Good pulp to pulp apposition for tripod pinch is the key to functional opposition and has been demonstrated to contribute significantly to improved Michigan Hand Questionnaire scores in our recent data analysis [19] (Fig. 6.2h). The donor foot deficit is demonstrated in these long-term follow-up photos, with no significant deficits noted on Foot Functional Index scores, and the patient did not require any walking aids or specialist footwear (Fig. 6.2i).

Case 2: Second Toe Wrap-Around Flap

The second toe wrap-around flap was described by Wei in 1991, primarily for partial finger defects involving degloving of the distal half of the fingers with intact bone and flexor digitorum superficialis tendon insertion [28]. As the skeleton is preserved, total range of motion (ROM) tends to be better than for a whole second toe (110° vs 65°) [17]. Here we illustrate this technique in a 30-year-old male patient who lost the tip of his left middle finger in 1992, following a failed attempt at replantation (Fig. 6.3a).

The finger defect was templated and transposed to the donor toe (Fig. 6.3b). A retrograde approach with a short pedicle technique was used—where the pedicle is taken either just short of the FDMA or with a small segment (Fig. 6.3c). The second toe wrap-around was taken with the distal phalanx, as this helps to prevent swivelling of the neo-fingertip on the degloved finger skeleton. The distal phalanx of the finger was shaped like a 'dowel' to allow fixation into a hole made in the base of the second toe distal phalanx. Aesthetic and functional results at 1 year (Fig. 6.3d–f) are shown, with accurate pulp to pulp apposition without instability.

Note that the donor toe was disarticulated through the MTP joint to allow primary closure, as this provides better aesthetic closure (Fig. 6.3g).

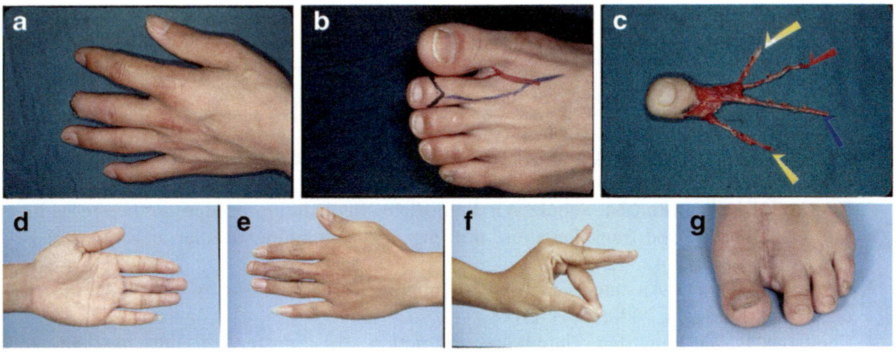

Fig. 6.3 Second toe wrap-around flap sequence of surgical steps (**a**–**g**)

Summary

Great and second toe transfers have transformed the management of traumatic and congenital thumb and finger absence, from early forays over a century ago until now, when large series of toe transfers now approach 100% success rates in specialist centres. Although strong validated outcome data exist for the efficacy of toe to thumb reconstruction, there are fewer data regarding its use for single-finger and particularly partial finger reconstruction. Future research centres around providing validated patient-reported outcome data that both supports the use of toe transfers over replantation or amputation and defines the relative strength of indications for toe transfer in different scenarios (single digit, multiple digits, isolated thumb, thumb and fingers, etc.) with greater clarity.

Key points to the dissection include the following:

- The first dorsal metatarsal artery is dominant in about 70–80% cases.
- Retrograde dissection of the vascular pedicle at the first webspace allows rapid identification of the dominant vessel, obviating the need to have an in-depth understanding of anatomical variations.
- Assiduous skeletonization of the vascular pedicles both provides a distal sympathectomy that reduces vasospasm risk and reduces bulk thereby allowing ease of passage of vessels through subcutaneous tunnels, especially in distal finger reconstruction.
- The proximal 1 cm of the proximal phalanx should be preserved when harvesting the great toe, preserving the windlass mechanism and function of the medial plantar arch. Recent data demonstrates normal foot outcomes when using validated patient-reported outcomes in comparison to control patients.
- If additional metacarpal length is required, either distraction osteogenesis or an iliac bone block and groin flap should be considered prior to great toe transfer.
- A first-stage groin flap should be considered when planning toe transfers, as it is preferable to augment soft tissue coverage instead of including too much skin from the foot. Skin grafts should be avoided in both the foot or the hand.

References

1. Buncke HJ, et al. Replantation surgery in China. Report of the American Replantation Mission to China. Plast Reconstr Surg. 1973;52(5):476–89.
2. Buncke HJ Jr, Buncke CM, Schulz WP. Immediate Nicoladoni procedure in the rhesus monkey, or hallux-to-hand transplantation, utilising microminiature vascular anastomoses. Br J Plast Surg. 1966;19(4):332–7.
3. Chung KC, Wei FC. An outcome study of thumb reconstruction using microvascular toe transfer. J Hand Surg Am. 2000;25(4):651–8.
4. Clarkson P, Furlong R. Thumb reconstruction by transfer of big toe. Br Med J. 1949;2(4640):1332–4, illust.

5. Cobbett JR. Free digital transfer. Report of a case of transfer of a great toe to replace an amputated thumb. J Bone Joint Surg Br. 1969;51(4):677–9.
6. Coskunfirat OK, Wei FC, Lin CH, Chen HC, Lin YT. Simultaneous double second toe transfer for reconstruction of adjacent fingers. Plast Reconstr Surg. 2005;115(4):1064–9.
7. del Piñal F. The indications for toe transfer after "minor" finger injuries. J Hand Surg Br. 2004;29(2):120–9.
8. Foucher G, Medina J, Navarro R, Nagel D. Toe transfer in congenital hand malformations. J Reconstr Microsurg. 2001;17(1):1–7.
9. Foucher G, Merle M, Maneaud M, Michon J. Microsurgical free partial toe transfer in hand reconstruction: a report of 12 cases. Plast Reconstr Surg. 1980;65(5):616–27.
10. Gabrielli C, Olave E. Origins of the dorsal metatarsal arteries in humans. Scand J Plast Reconstr Surg Hand Surg. 2002;36(4):221–5.
11. Gilbert A. Composite tissue transfers from the foot: anatomic basis and surgical technique. In: Symposium on Microsurgery. S. B. Daniller A. St Louis, Mo, Mosby; 1976.
12. Henry SL, Wei FC. Thumb reconstruction with toe transfer. J Hand Microsurg. 2010;2(2):72–8.
13. Hou Z, Zou J, Wang Z, Zhong S. Anatomical classification of the first dorsal metatarsal artery and its clinical application. Plast Reconstr Surg. 2013;132(6):1028e–39e.
14. Kay SP, Wiberg M. Toe to hand transfer in children. Part 1: technical aspects. J Hand Surg Br. 1996;21(6):723–34.
15. Kay SP, Wiberg M, Bellew M, Webb F. Toe to hand transfer in children. Part 2: functional and psychological aspects. J Hand Surg Br. 1996;21(6):735–45.
16. Kotkansalo T, Vilkki S, Elo P. Long-term results of finger reconstruction with microvascular toe transfers after trauma. J Plast Reconstr Aesthet Surg. 2011;64(10):1291–9.
17. Lin PY, Sebastin SJ, Ono S, Bellfi LT, Chang KW, Chung KC. A systematic review of outcomes of toe-to-thumb transfers for isolated traumatic thumb amputation. Hand (N Y). 2011;6(3):235–43.
18. Lin YT, Loh CYY, Lien SH, Lin CH, Wei FC. Simultaneous Stiles-Bunnell tendon transfer enhances intrinsic function of second-toe transplantations. Plast Reconstr Surg. 2017;140(6):1229–34.
19. Lo S, Wei FC. Toe transfers outperform replantation after digit amputations: outcomes of 126 toe transfers. Plast Reconstr Surg. 2025;156(2):267–77. https://doi.org/10.1097/PRS.0000000000012053.
20. Nguyen VT, Lam K, Le VD. Using 320-detector row computed tomography angiography to investigate the arterial anatomy of the toe flaps on living humans. Surg Radiol Anat. 2021;43(10):1711–9.
21. Nicoladoni C. Daumenplastik. Wien Klin Wochenschr. 1897;28:663–6.
22. Nikkhah D, Martin N, Pickford M. Paediatric toe-to-hand transfer: an assessment of outcomes from a single unit. J Hand Surg Eur. 2016;41(3):281–94.
23. Ntuli S, Nalla S, Kiter A. Anatomical variation of the dorsalis pedis artery in a South African population - a cadaveric study. Foot (Edinb). 2018;35:16–27.
24. Swanson AB, Göran-Hagert C, de Groot Swanson G. Evaluation of impairment in the upper extremity. J Hand Surg Am. 1987;12(5 Pt 2):896–926.
25. Tang SFT, Tang ACW, Chen CK, Wu HM, Wei FC. Foot plantar pressure profile alteration after microsurgical great toe-to-thumb transfer. Plast Reconstr Surg Glob Open. 2023;11(9):e5228.
26. Wei FC, Chen HC, Chuang CC, Chen SH. Microsurgical thumb reconstruction with toe transfer: selection of various techniques. Plast Reconstr Surg. 1994;93(2):345-351; discussion 352-347.
27. Wei FC, Chen HC, Chuang CC, Noordhoff MS. Simultaneous multiple toe transfers in hand reconstruction. Plast Reconstr Surg. 1988;81(3):366–77.
28. Wei FC, Chen HC, Chuang DC, Chen S, Noordhoff MS. Second toe wrap-around flap. Plast Reconstr Surg. 1991;88(5):837–43.

29. Wei FC, Colony LH, Chen HC, Chuang CC, Noordhoff MS. Combined second and third toe transfer. Plast Reconstr Surg. 1989;84(4):651–61.
30. Wei FC, el-Gammal TA, Lin CH, Chuang CC, Chen HC, Chen SH. Metacarpal hand: classification and guidelines for microsurgical reconstruction with toe transfers. Plast Reconstr Surg. 1997;99(1):122–8.
31. Wei FC, Epstein MD, Chen HC, Chuang CC, Chen HT. Microsurgical reconstruction of distal digits following mutilating hand injuries: results in 121 patients. Br J Plast Surg. 1993;46(3):181–6.
32. Wei FC, Silverman RT, Hsu WM. Retrograde dissection of the vascular pedicle in toe harvest. Plast Reconstr Surg. 1995;96(5):1211–4.
33. Wei FC, Yim KK. Pulp plasty after toe-to-hand transplantation. Plast Reconstr Surg. 1995;96(3):661–6.
34. Zhu J, Hu B. Sonography of the first dorsal metatarsal artery of the foot. J Clin Ultrasound. 2006;34(1):1–4.

Chapter 7
"Other" Donor Sites for Vascularized Bone Transfer from the Foot

Jenny Lee Nguyen and William C. Pederson

The primary donor sites for vascularized bone transfer from the foot are the toes for reconstruction of the loss of a thumb or finger(s). Microsurgical toe transfer has proven to be a reliable and very functional transfer in experienced hands. Both the great toe and second and/or third toe can be harvested based on the dorsal and volar circulation. The great toe is generally utilized for thumb reconstruction and the secondary toes utilized for finger reconstruction [12]. Many variations of toe transfers exist, including double toe transfer, partial toe transfer, and "wraparound" transfer of the great toe (Fig. 7.1). One obviously needs to be aware of the morbidity of these transfers, but in general they are well-tolerated and the trade-off of morbidity in the foot is generally thought to be reasonable based on the improvement in hand function. These will be described fully in another chapter.

Other bones which may be transferred are the metatarsal(s) and various modifications of toe bone and joint transfers. This chapter will discuss these alternative options and vascular anatomy of these potential donor sites. Again, we are always weighing the morbidity in the foot vs. the improvement in function in the hand or wherever the bone may be transferred.

J. L. Nguyen
Texas Children's Hospital and Baylor College of Medicine, Houston, TX, USA
e-mail: JennyLee.Nguyen@bcm.edu

W. C. Pederson (✉)
Josephine Abercrombie Endowed Professor of Plastic Surgery, Baylor College of Medicine and Texas Children's Hospital, Houston, TX, USA

Surgery, Orthopedic Surgery, Neurosurgery, and Pediatrics, Baylor College of Medicine, Houston, TX, USA
e-mail: wcpeders@texaschildrens.org

J. P. Agarwal, D. W. Mathes (eds.), *Bone Flaps in Reconstructive Surgery*,
https://doi.org/10.1007/978-3-032-12540-8_7

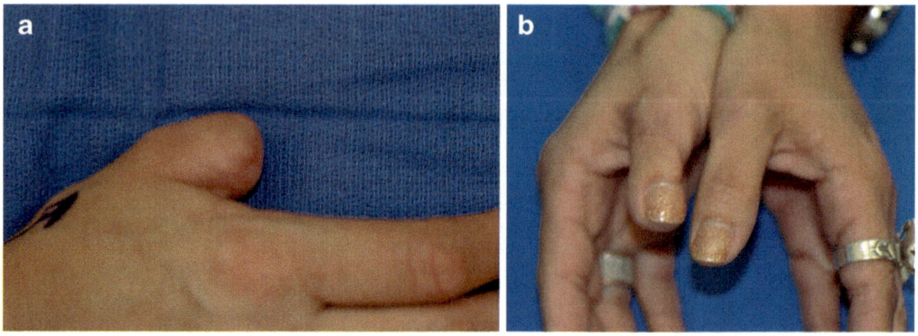

Fig. 7.1 (**a**) Pre-op view of 39 y/o female after loss of right thumb. (**b**) 6-month post-op view after great toe wraparound flap side to side with opposite thumb.

Metatarsal Transfer

The first, second, and potentially the third metatarsals may be transferred, with or without skin (the dorsalis pedis flap) and either the proximal or distal joints (metatarsophalangeal [MTP] and/or tarsometatarsal [TMT] joints). The first and second metatarsals are based primarily on the dorsalis pedis artery running either dorsally or in the deep webspace between the first and second metatarsal. This vascular anatomy was classically described by Gilbert, who found three primary variations [7]. In Type I, the first dorsal metatarsal artery runs on top of the fascia in the first interspace, in Type II the artery runs in the interosseous muscles, and in Type III the artery is found plantar to the interspace and muscles. More recently, Hou and colleagues studied this anatomy and found that the artery was never entirely in the muscle, but rather between the muscle and the first metatarsal [8]. This finding, however, is not totally inconsistent with the findings of Gilbert.

It would be unusual to take both the first and second metatarsals due to potential morbidity in the foot. For reconstruction of intercalated gaps in the bony skeletons of the thumb or fingers, the second metatarsal and MTP joint can be utilized to good effect with or without the second toe. In general, the great toe would not be harvested with the first metatarsal due to potential morbidity of the foot. With loss of the first metacarpal in the hand and/or the thumb, the second metatarsal and second toe present a nearly ideal reconstruction, pollicization notwithstanding. Likewise, with partial loss of the metacarpal and maintenance of the thumb intact, the second metatarsal can give an ideal reconstruction. The issue of reconstruction of the first carpometacarpal joint of the hand does not have any great solution, but the proximal metatarsal can be fused to the remaining carpus or alternatively tied down with suture, allowing some motion. It is unclear which is superior, but a fixed thumb metacarpal can be quite functional (but does not allow the patient to lay the hand flat on a surface) (Fig. 7.2).

Del Pinal has utilized the *base* of the third metatarsal with its cartilage as a vascularized graft to reconstruct the distal radioulnar joint (DRUJ) and some of the

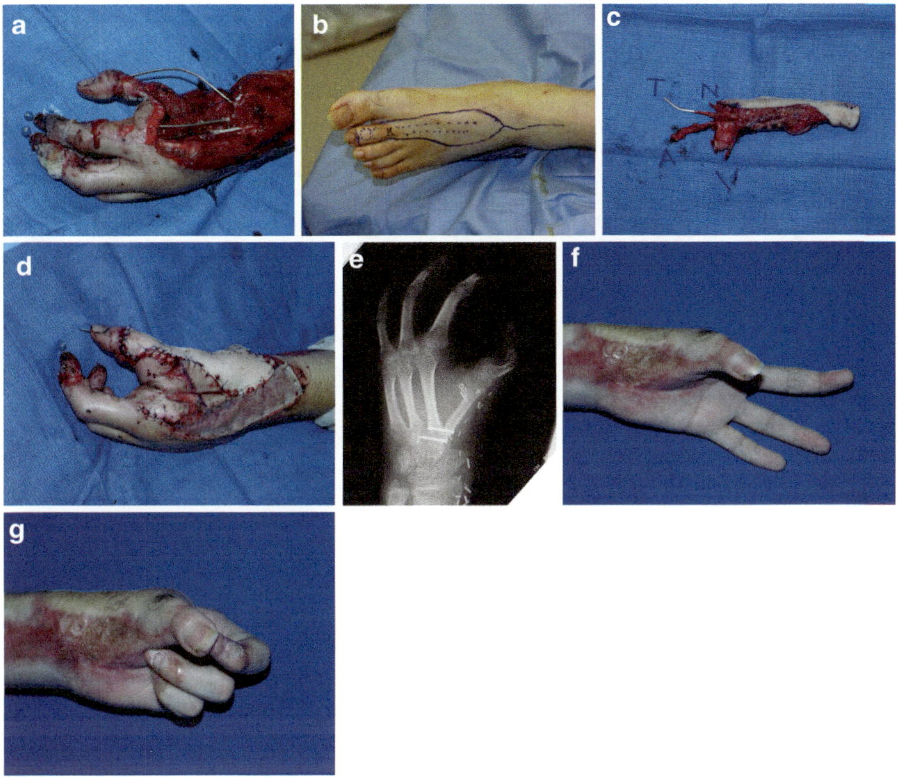

Fig. 7.2 (**a**) View of 18 y/o male's hand after rollover MVA. Note absence of first and second metacarpal and proximal phalanx of thumb. (**b**) Flap containing second metatarsal, proximal phalanx of second toe, and dorsalis pedis soft tissue flap based on the dorsalis pedis artery. (**c**) View of flap on back towel with tendons and vessels marked. (**d**) Flap inset into hand to replace the first metacarpal and proximal phalanx of the thumb. (**e**) X-Ray at 6 months. (**f**) Thumb extension at 6 months. (**g**) Thumb flexion at 6 months

radial articular surface [3, 5]. We do not have any experience with this technique, but the dissection is reportedly quite difficult and the morbidity, while reportedly low, is a bit unclear. This is certainly an innovative way to attempt reconstruction of an otherwise nearly impossible defect.

Vascularized Toe Joint Transfer

Vascularized toe joint transfer has been performed for many years. This has utilized both the MTP joint (for the hand MCP joints) [10] and the interphalangeal joint (for the proximal interphalangeal joints) [18]. The application of these two vascularized bone transfers for digital reconstruction has been somewhat limited as other options

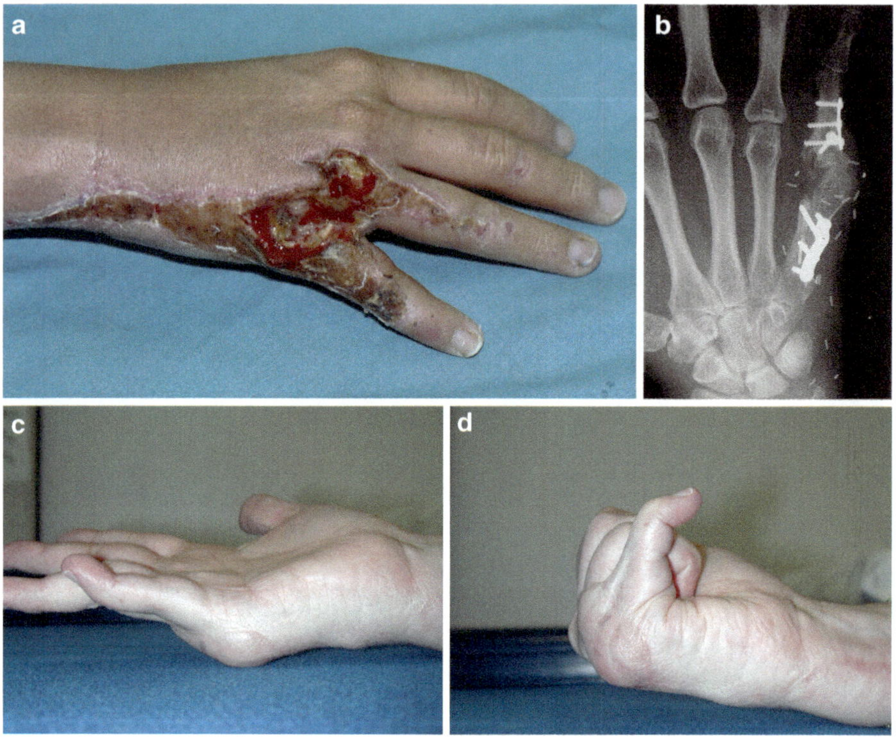

Fig. 7.3 (**a**) View of 23 y/o female piano teacher after rollover motor vehicle accident. The fifth MCP joint has been ground off. (**b**) 15-year follow-up X-ray showing "upside-down" position of the foot MTP joint. (**c**) 15-year follow-up, extension. (**d**) 15-year follow-up, flexion

usually exist. The transfer can be technically difficult, and in the MCP position, the MTP joint from the foot needs to be turned around 180° (dorsal-volarly) in order to have the appropriate range of motion [10]. While results can be quite good, long-term studies have shown that motion is usually limited to around 35–50°, and thus, vascularized toe joint transfers are done rather infrequently (Fig. 7.3).

Other Applications of Second MTP Joint Transfers

Vilkki, notably, has utilized the second MTP joint of the toe for a number of applications besides digital reconstruction [14]. He has written extensively on using this vascularized joint in children with the physis as a management for radial longitudinal deficiency [15]. In this technique, the proximal metatarsal is inserted into the distal ulna and the proximal phalanx of the toe is attached to the more radial carpus. While this has the potential for growth, even Vilkki's own studies have shown that the toe physis often does not keep up with growth of the distal ulna, leading to poor correction of the deformity. His most recent report addressed this and other issues with this transfer with some improvement in results [17].

Besides application in radial longitudinal deficiency, he has also done cadaver studies using the metatarsal head to reconstruct a "neolunate" in cases of Keinbock's [16]. The long-term results of this transfer are not clear at this point. Cavadas from Spain has utilized two MTP joints to reconstruct destroyed radiocarpal joints in two patients. He reports that good range of motion and pain control were present 4 years post-op [1]. Del Pinal recently reported the use of the MTP joint to reconstruct the scaphotrapezial joint after distal scaphoid excision and carpal collapse. His report states that at 3 years post-op the patient had normal range of motion and no pain [2]. All of these reports emphasize the utility of the second MTP joint for reconstruction of small joints of the hand and wrist. These procedures, however, can be technically demanding and are rarely indicated in most hands.

Partial Toe Joint Transfers

The next area of consideration is the use of portions of the toe joints for reconstruction of various joint surface defects in the hand. The use of hemi-toe joint transfers has been proposed in certain circumstances, and though there are few reports of this, it may be a reasonable approach in certain instances.

The second metatarsal with the head and proximal joint surface has been utilized for a number of different reconstructions. Our group studied the anatomy of the second metatarsal head and collateral ligaments and found that the curve of the metatarsal head could closely match the curve of the same individual's scaphoid [11], but have not had the opportunity to apply this finding in a patient. Del Pinal has utilized a vascularized metatarsal head for reconstruction of the ulnar head after traumatic loss [4]. At 4-year follow-up, the patient was pain-free but with somewhat limited pronation and supination. The favorable shape of the metatarsal head has also been utilized to reconstruct the metacarpal head in the face of osteomyelitis [9]. Likewise, this graft has been utilized to stabilize an unstable congenital thumb with a Blauth-IIIB-type hypoplasia [6].

We reported a case of reconstruction of the lunate fossa of the distal radius using the proximal articular surface of the great toe proximal phalanx [13]. This patient had an excellent result for an otherwise extremely difficult problem which allowed him to have continued motion with minimal pain (Fig. 7.4). All of these partial transfers are complex surgical procedures and have limited application, but can provide articular surface and/or ligaments for reconstruction of small joints in the hand.

The foot, while offering rather limited donor material, can offer several options for vascularized bone transfer which are not available elsewhere in the body. These can be utilized to reconstruct some defects that present difficult challenges for the reconstructive surgeon. Regardless, the surgeon must always be aware of the potential morbidity of these donor sites and select their usage accordingly.

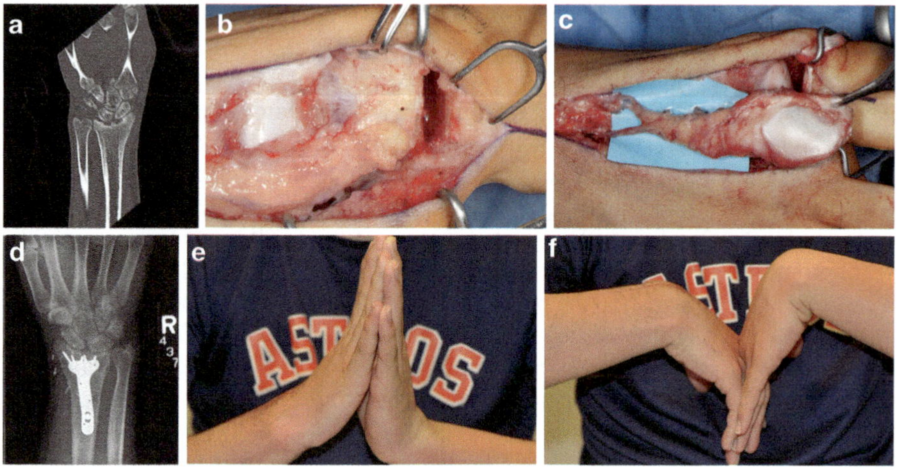

Fig. 7.4 (**a**) CT scan of 18 y/o male 6 months after fall from horse. (**b**) View of MTP joint and proximal phalanx of the toe. The pedicle to proximal portion of the proximal phalanx is below. Osteotomy of the mid-proximal phalanx is to the right. (**c**) View of the articular surface of the proximal phalanx of the great toe on the vascular pedicle prior to placement in scaphoid fossa for reconstruction of joint surface. (**d**) 8-month post-op view of distal radius and radiocarpal joint. (**e**) Dorsiflexion (right hand) at 8 months. (**f**) Palmar flexion (right hand) at 8 months

References

1. Cavadas PC, Padial B. Radiocarpal joint reconstruction with a double free metatarsophalangeal joint transfer. Plast Reconstr Surg Glob Open. 2023;11(9). https://doi.org/10.1097/GOX.0000000000005284.
2. del Piñal F, Cromheecke M, Chaves C. Free vascularized second metatarsophalangeal joint transfer for scaphotrapezial joint reconstruction after distal scaphoid excision and carpal collapse: a case report. Microsurgery. 2022;42(3). https://doi.org/10.1002/micr.30835.
3. Del Piñal F, García-Bernal FJ, Delgado J, Sanmartín M, Regalado J. Reconstruction of the distal radius facet by a free vascularized osteochondral autograft: anatomic study and report of a patient. J Hand Surg. 2005;30(6). https://doi.org/10.1016/j.jhsa.2005.07.005.
4. Del Piñal F, Guerrero-Navarro ML, Studer A, Thams C, Moraleda E. Reconstruction of the ulnar head with a vascularized second metatarsal head: case report. J Hand Surg. 2012;37(8). https://doi.org/10.1016/j.jhsa.2012.04.039.
5. Del Piñal F, Klausmeyer M, Moraleda E, De Piero GH, Galindo C, Studer A, Cerezal L. Vascularized graft from the metatarsal base for reconstructing major osteochondral distal radius defects. J Hand Surg. 2013;38(10). https://doi.org/10.1016/j.jhsa.2013.07.013.
6. Fang X, Yu A, Dai X, Bai H, Zhou J, Li D, Du X, Tian J, Zhou S, Wang B. Reconstruction of type IIIB thumb hypoplasia using a vascularized hemi-metatarsal composite tissue flap. Plast Reconstr Surg. 2023;152(5). https://doi.org/10.1097/PRS.0000000000010513.
7. Gilbert A. Reconstruction of congenital hand defects with microvascular toe transfers. Hand Clin. 1985;1(2). https://doi.org/10.1016/s0749-0712(21)01361-5.
8. Hou Z, Zou J, Wang Z, Zhong S. Anatomical classification of the first dorsal metatarsal artery and its clinical application. Plast Reconstr Surg. 2013;132(6). https://doi.org/10.1097/PRS.0b013e3182a97de6.

9. Isenberg JS. Additional experience with hemi-metatarsal vascularized bone transfer for treatment of phalangeal osteomyelitis. J Reconstr Microsurg. 2000;16(7). https://doi.org/10.1055/s-2000-8393.
10. Kanaya K, Wada T, Usui M, Yamashita T. Fourteen-year results of a reversed vascularized second metatarsophalangeal joint transfer: a case report. J Hand Surg. 2005;30(1). https://doi.org/10.1016/j.jhsa.2004.08.008.
11. Larkins CG, Tannan SC, Burkett AE, Mithani SK, Srinivasan RC, Pederson WC. Autologous osteoligamentous reconstruction of scaphoid proximal pole with metatarsal head and collateral ligament: cadaver anatomic description of novel surgical technique. Hand. 2021;16(6). https://doi.org/10.1177/1558944719895616.
12. Lin PY, Sebastin SJ, Ono S, Bellfi LT, Chang KWC, Chung KC. A systematic review of outcomes of toe-to-thumb transfers for isolated traumatic thumb amputation. Hand. 2011;6(3). https://doi.org/10.1007/s11552-011-9340-x.
13. Pederson WC, Killion E, White L. Reconstruction of a portion of the articular surface of the distal radius with a vascularized Osteochondral graft from the proximal phalanx of the great toe. J Hand Surg Glob Online. 2021;3(4). https://doi.org/10.1016/j.jhsg.2021.04.002.
14. Vilkki S. Microsurgical MTP. Hand. 2016;11(1_suppl). https://doi.org/10.1177/1558944716660555ek.
15. Vilkki SK. Distraction and microvascular epiphysis transfer for radial club hand. J Hand Surg: Eur Vol. 1998;23(4). https://doi.org/10.1016/S0266-7681(98)80120-4.
16. Vilkki SK. A new concept and technique for custom-made microvascular lunate bone reconstruction. J Reconstr Microsurg. 2007;23(7). https://doi.org/10.1055/s-2007-992335.
17. Vilkki SK, Paavilainen P. Vascularized second metatarsophalangeal joint transfer for radial deficiency – an update. J Hand Surg (Eur Vol). 2018;43(9). https://doi.org/10.1177/1753193418793597.
18. Zhou KJ, Graham DJ, Lawson RD, Sivakumar BS. Toe-to-finger vascularized joint transfers for proximal interphalangeal joint reconstruction: a systematic review. Hand. 2022;17(6). https://doi.org/10.1177/1558944720988081.

Chapter 8
Iliac Crest Flap

Z-Hye Lee and Matthew M. Hanasono

Introduction

The iliac crest flap, also known as the deep circumflex iliac artery (DCIA) flap, is a versatile option that provides high-quality vascularized bone and additional soft tissue components. The bone has a robust blood supply including both nutrient and periosteal perforators which allows for longitudinal splitting and osteotomies to appropriately contour the bone. First described by Taylor et al. [1] in 1979, the traditional flap included iliac crest bone, a substantial amount of abdominal musculature, and overlying skin. However, the flap as originally described has several disadvantages including excess bulk due to inclusion of the abdominal muscles, an unreliable skin paddle, and donor site morbidity arising from detachment of abdominal and thigh muscles from the iliac crest. Several refinements were developed in recent decades to address these problems [2]. Safak et al. [3] identified musculocutaneous perforators that could be isolated to perfuse the skin paddle without including a large muscle cuff. Several years later, Shenaq et al. [4] modified the design of the bone harvest to include only the inner cortex and leaving the outer cortex with the thigh muscle attachments intact. More recent studies have mapped the exact anatomy of perforators arising from the deep circumflex iliac artery (DCIA) allowing for greater mobility of the skin component and reducing the overall soft tissue volume. With these modifications, the iliac crest flap is an excellent osteocutaneous reconstructive flap option and valid alternative for patients with arterial disease or abnormal lower limb anatomy in whom a fibula flap is contraindicated.

Z.-H. Lee · M. M. Hanasono (✉)
Department of Plastic Surgery, The University of Texas MD Anderson Cancer Center, Houston, TX, USA
e-mail: mhanasono@mdanderson.org

J. P. Agarwal, D. W. Mathes (eds.), *Bone Flaps in Reconstructive Surgery*,
https://doi.org/10.1007/978-3-032-12540-8_8

Indications

The iliac crest flap is an excellent choice in the head and neck region for reconstruction of both the mandible and the maxilla [5]. For mandibular reconstruction, the ipsilateral iliac crest flap is typically chosen so that the reconstruction plate can be fixated to the outer surface of the bone which faces extraorally and the inner surface of the bone with the pedicle faces intraorally (Fig. 8.1). The iliac crest bone has a natural curvature that corresponds almost exactly to the maxilla and the height and depth of this bone can provide excellent facial contour for a total maxillectomy defect [6]. The internal oblique muscle or the skin paddle can be used to reconstruct the nasal and oral cavity. In addition, the generous cortical bone stock allows for placement of osseointegrated dental implants in both mandibular and maxillary reconstruction. This flap can also be used for long-bone reconstruction such as for the tibia although its natural curvature does not provide a straight segment of bone longer than 10 cm. While this flap is most commonly used as a free flap, pedicled vascularized iliac crest flaps have been described for hip reconstruction in defects involving the acetabulum [7].

Despite these advantages, it should be noted that the iliac crest may also have some limitations. Even when harvested as a perforator flap, the associated skin paddle can be quite thick in some patients, which may be less ideal for intraoral resurfacing. In these scenarios, a second flap such as a fasciocutaneous forearm flap may be required if thin soft tissue coverage is needed. In addition, the pedicle length is relatively short especially when compared to the fibula free flap which may pose challenges, particularly in maxillary reconstruction. Either vein grafts or an intraoral approach with anastomoses to the facial artery and vein may be required [8]. It is also important to note that iliac crest flap dissection can be difficult and

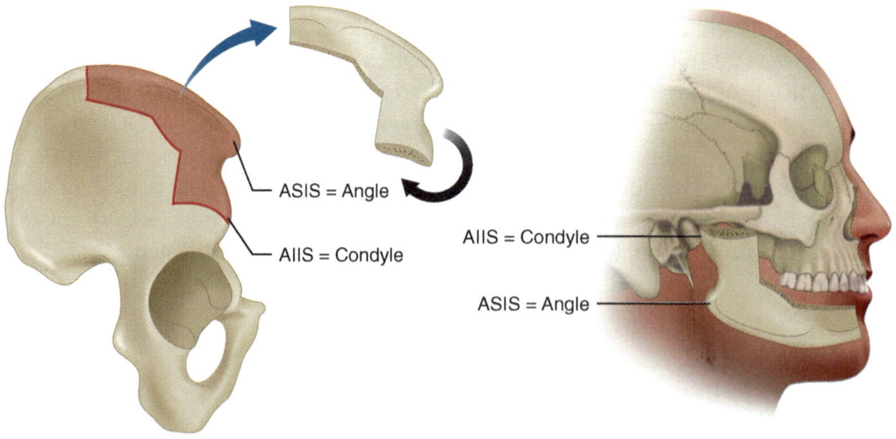

Fig. 8.1 The ipsilateral iliac crest may be used to reconstruct a hemimandibular defect. The anterior superior iliac spine becomes the angle of the mandible and the natural curvature of the iliac crest mimics the curvature of the mandible such that shaping osteotomies are usually not necessary

sometimes unfeasible in obese patients. Patients with previous abdominal or inguinal surgery may not be suitable candidates given that there may be damage or fibrosis affecting the pedicle. It is because of these relative disadvantages that the iliac crest flap is often considered a second-line option behind the fibula free flap in osseous and osteocutaneous head and neck reconstruction.

Anatomy

In most cases, the deep circumflex iliac artery (DCIA) blood supply arises from the posterolateral side of the external iliac artery at the level of the inguinal ligament (Fig. 8.2). In some cases, it can also arise from the femoral artery slightly below the inguinal ligament [9]. The deep inferior epigastric vessels originate from a similar location on the external iliac vessels but course medially. Originating deep to the transversalis fascia, the DCIA then travels superolaterally towards the anterior superior iliac spine (ASIS). Within 1 cm of the ASIS, it gives rise to a large ascending branch or several smaller branches that nourish the internal oblique muscle which

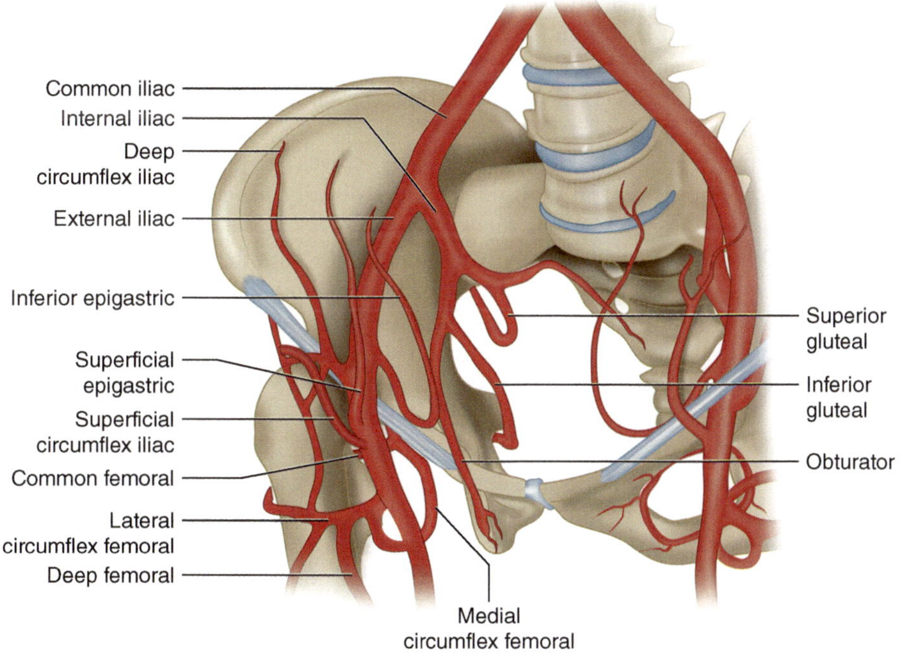

Fig. 8.2 Vascular anatomy in the region of the ilium. The deep circumflex iliac artery (DCIA) usually arises from the external iliac artery at about the same level as the deep inferior epigastric, just before the artery crosses the inguinal ligament and becomes known as the common femoral artery

can be included with this flap [10]. These branches penetrate the transversalis fascia and travel in between the internal oblique and transversus abdominis muscles before anastomosing with the deep inferior epigastric artery.

The main transverse branch of DCIA continues laterally along the inner (deep) surface of the iliac crest in a fibro-osseous tunnel between the insertion of the transversus abdominis and internal oblique muscles. During this course, the DCIA gives several small periosteal perforators that supply the medial surface of the iliac crest. In addition, several musculocutaneous perforators pass through the transversus abdominis, internal oblique, and external oblique muscles to the overlying skin [11]. These perforators are almost always present, but their size and location can be variable. Taylor et al. [1] demonstrated an average of six musculocutaneous perforators, while Safak et al. [3] found a cluster of musculocutaneous perforators in 70% of cadaver dissections and a single dominant perforator in 30%. Bergeron et al. [12] demonstrated that the average number of DCIA perforators was 1.6 (range 0–5) and were most commonly located 5 to 10 cm (average 7.4 cm) lateral to the ASIS and located 0.1 to 3.5 cm (average 0.8 cm) above the iliac crest bone. A handheld Doppler is useful to identify the position of dominant perforators and properly position the skin island. The main DCIA then emerges from the fibro-osseous tunnel posteriorly and pierces the transversus abdominis muscle to anastomose with the lumbar and/or iliolumbar arteries.

The iliac crest flap typically has a pedicle length of about 5 to 7 cm with a diameter of 1.5 to 2 mm at its origin [13]. There are typically two deep circumflex iliac veins that converge at the level of the inguinal ligament to form a single vein. This deep circumflex iliac vein (DCIV) crosses the external iliac artery either in front or behind to drain into the external iliac vein.

The superficial circumflex iliac artery (SCIA) serves as a minor blood supply to the iliac crest bone. It typically originates more distally from the femoral vessels and supplies the skin anterior and superior to the ASIS as well as an osseous segment laterally near the ASIS. It usually communicates with the DCIA in the region of the iliac crest and can be used to support a larger skin paddle.

While the flap is not sensate and no motor nerves travel with the pedicle, several important sensory nerves in the groin region should be preserved during flap harvest. In the groin between the external iliac vessels and the ASIS, the lateral femoral cutaneous nerve lies lateral to the ilioinguinal nerve. It travels through or inferior to the inguinal ligament approximately, sometimes piercing the sartorius muscle, about 1 cm medial to the ASIS and descends along a line connecting the ASIS and the superolateral corner of the patella. Entrapment of this nerve may cause pain in the thigh and groin, a condition known as meralgia paresthetica. Division of the nerve will result in permanent numbness in the anterolateral thigh. The ilioinguinal nerve (L1) travels between the internal and external oblique muscles and can be encountered inferior to the pedicle as it travels towards the ASIS. It travels along the spermatic cord and provides innervation to the proximal medial thigh and the perineal region. The iliohypogastric nerve travels between the transversus abdominis and internal oblique layers of the abdominal wall and can be encountered superior to the pedicle and medial to the ASIS.

Operative Technique

The flap is harvested with the patient in supine position. A roll is placed under the contralateral hip to improve exposure while dissecting within the iliac fossa. The skin paddle is marked two-thirds above and one-third below the line of the anterior iliac crest. The skin paddle can measure 15 to 20 cm in length and 6 to 8 cm in width depending on skin laxity (Fig. 8.3). The skin incision is extended medially about 1 cm superior to the inguinal ligament, towards the inguinal canal, to identify the pedicle and begin flap harvest. The superficial inguinal ring and round ligament or spermatic cord are identified and retracted medially. The transversalis fascia is incised to expose the external iliac artery and vein which are dissected to identify the DCIA and DCIV. All the layers of the abdominal musculature including the external oblique, internal oblique, and transversus abdominis are divided from the inguinal ligament to expose the pedicle. The pedicle is then dissected laterally towards the ASIS. The ascending branch is then encountered about 1 cm medial to the ASIS adherent to the deep surface of the internal oblique muscle. If needed, this

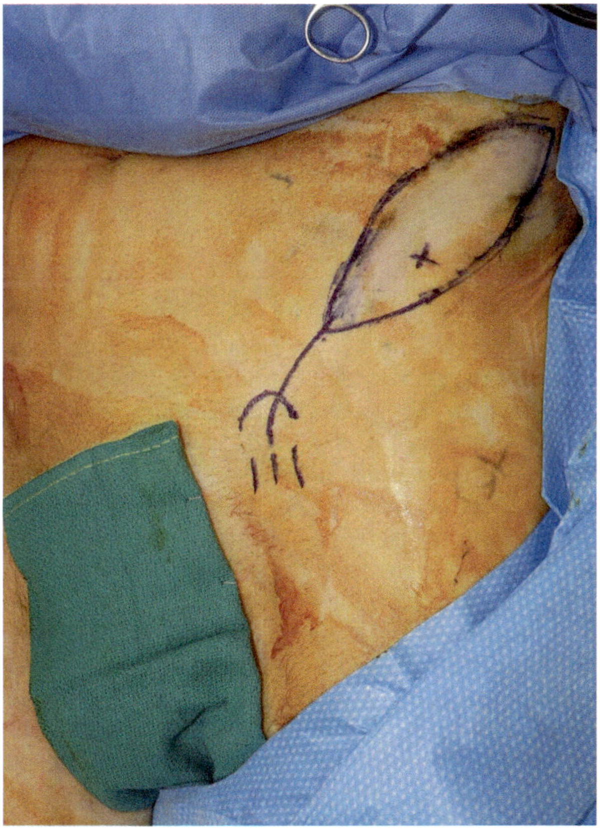

Fig. 8.3 Skin markings for a left iliac crest osteocutaneous free flap. The skin paddle has been marked and is centered over the superior margin of the ilium. An incision will be made over the inguinal ligament extending inferiorly to the inguinal ring

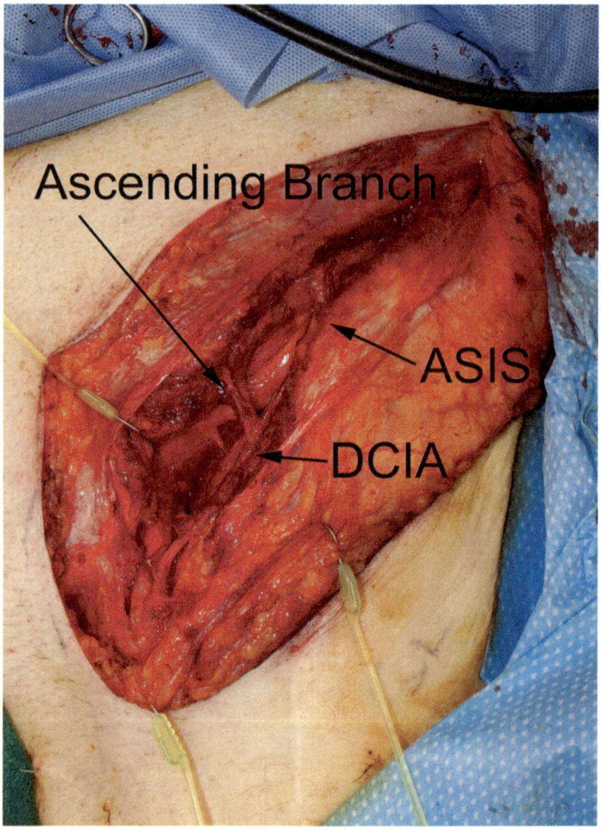

Fig. 8.4 Exposure of the deep circumflex iliac artery (DCIA) pedicle. The ascending branch has been dissected medial to the anterior superior iliac spine (ASIS). The external oblique, internal oblique, and transversus abdominis muscles have been divided from the inguinal ligament and superior margin of the ilium

branch can be used to harvest a segment of internal oblique muscle (Fig. 8.4). Otherwise, it is ligated and divided.

The skin incision is extended laterally and superiorly along the intended superior aspect of the skin paddle. Suprafascial dissection is performed inferiorly towards the iliac crest until perforators are encountered at which point the external oblique fascia is divided. It is important to note that perforators to the skin at this location can come from multiple sources including the intercostal vessels, lumbar vessels, or deep circumflex iliac vessels. Therefore, the perforators should be traced proximally to ensure that they originate from the DCIA. These typically do not have an associated nerve and have a more anterior orientation, while perforators originating from the intercostal or iliolumbar vessels usually have a nerve associated with them. If there is a single dominant perforator of 1 mm or greater in diameter, the skin paddle can be harvested as a true perforator-based flap to minimize bulk (Fig. 8.5). If there are multiple small perforators, a cuff of muscle should be included incorporating all of the perforators to ensure adequate perfusion.

The preperitoneal fat is retracted medially and superiorly to expose the iliacus muscle and fascia. The pedicle lies adherent to the inner cortex of the iliac crest

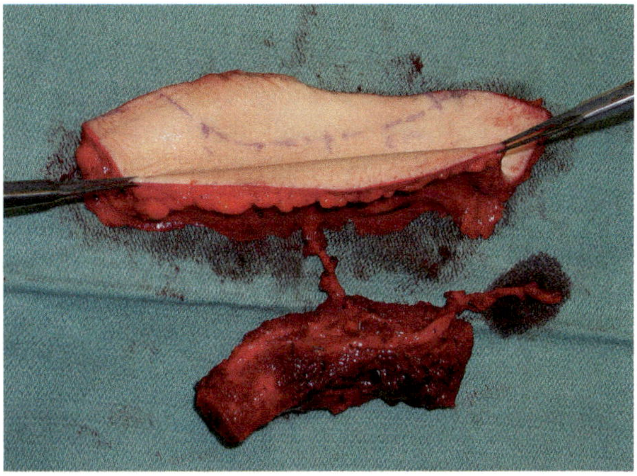

Fig. 8.5 Fully dissected iliac crest flap with a single perforator dissected to supply a skin paddle. The DCIA pedicle is visible entering the flap on the right side

bone within a fibro-osseous tunnel between the overhanging transversus muscle and the iliacus muscle. The iliacus muscle is divided from the iliac bone, exposing the fibro-osseous inner surface of the ilium. Next, the lower incision of the intended skin paddle is made and suprafascial dissection is performed cranially towards the iliac crest. If a harvest of full-thickness iliac crest bone is planned, the thigh muscle attachments are released from the outer (superficial) iliac crest, and the inguinal ligament is detached from the ASIS. However, this type of harvest carries a higher risk of abdominal hernia formation and gait disturbance. Alternately, only the inner cortex with a rim of iliac crest bone may be harvested to avoid detaching the thigh muscle attachments. In this case, the periosteum of the outer rim of the iliac crest is stripped for about 1 cm with minimal disturbance of the thigh muscle and tendon attachments. A segment of bone measuring up to 4 cm in height and 16 cm in length can be harvested. The appropriate bone dimensions are marked, and osteotomies are completed with an oscillating saw. We prefer to make osteotomies from the outer (superficial) cortex when harvesting a full-thickness bone flap. For an inner cortex-only flap, osteotomies are taken from the inner (deep) cortex and then the bone is split by making osteotomies along the superior edge of the iliac crest and extending the cuts with an oscillating saw or osteotome through the medullary bone. Virtual surgical planning guides can also be placed to help guide the bony cuts at this stage. Bone wax is used to aid with hemostasis along all bleeding bone surfaces.

Meticulous donor site closure is crucial to minimize abdominal hernia and gait issues. The iliacus and transversus muscle layers are reapproximated to the inner table of the iliac bone. Drill holes through the iliac bone may be necessary to appropriately anchor the muscles. Patients may benefit from mesh reinforcement of the closure (we prefer a 3–4-mm thick bioprosthetic mesh). Next, the hip is flexed, and the external oblique muscle is sutured to the upper thigh muscle attachments and periosteum. Strong, permanent sutures such as #1 polypropylene should be used. Closed suction drains are recommended to prevent seromas.

Case Example

A 70-year-old male had a history of carcinoma of the left maxilla treated by surgery and radiation. He subsequently developed osteoradionecrosis (ORN) of the left mandible with a draining orocutaneous fistula. He underwent segmental mandibulectomy from the left angle of the mandible to the left parasymphysis (Fig. 8.6). An iliac crest free flap was selected for reconstruction of the mandibular defect. Because the abdominal pannus was excessively thick for oral cavity reconstruction and there was a through and through soft tissue defect extending from the left floor of the mouth and gingiva to the left neck along the fistula tract, a separate soft tissue free flap was planned for reconstruction.

Computer-aided design and computer-aided manufacturing (CAD/CAM) was used to plan the surgery and fabricate computer-generated mandibular and iliac bone cutting guides (Fig. 8.7). A left iliac crest osseous free flap was harvested as described above (Fig. 8.8). For the intraoral and external soft tissue defects, an

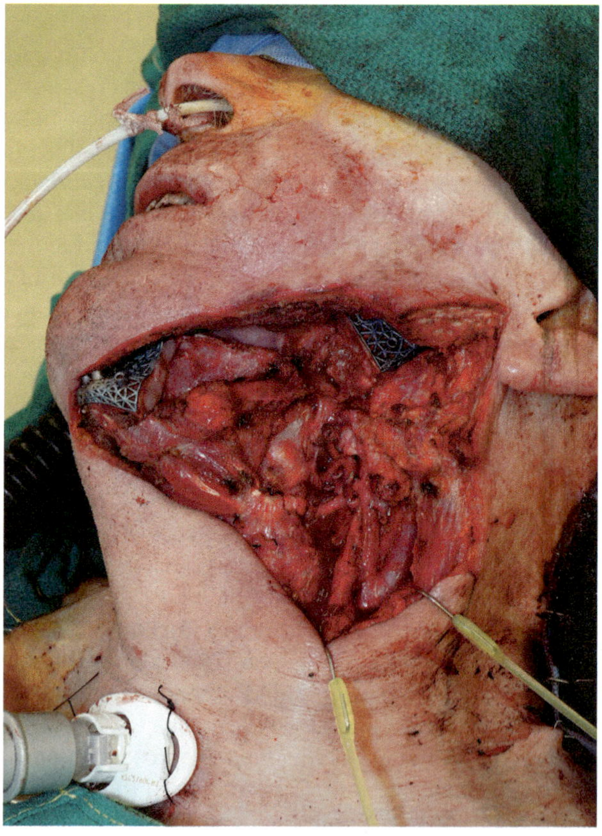

Fig. 8.6 A segmental mandibulectomy defect from the left angle of the mandible to the left parasymphysis

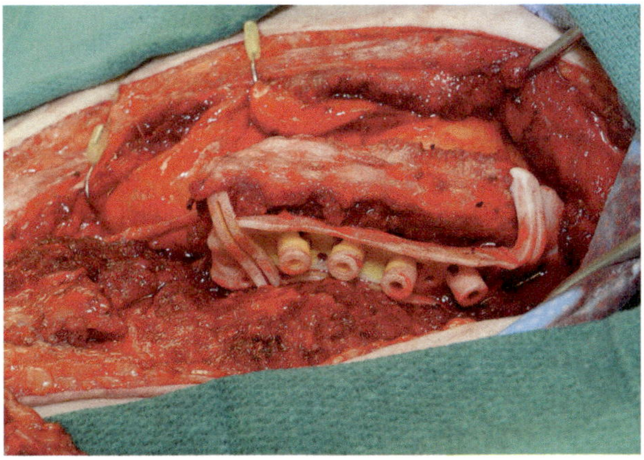

Fig. 8.7 A computer-generated 3D printed cutting guide is used to assist with making osteotomies on the left iliac crest as well as drill holes for screws used for rigid fixation to a titanium plate

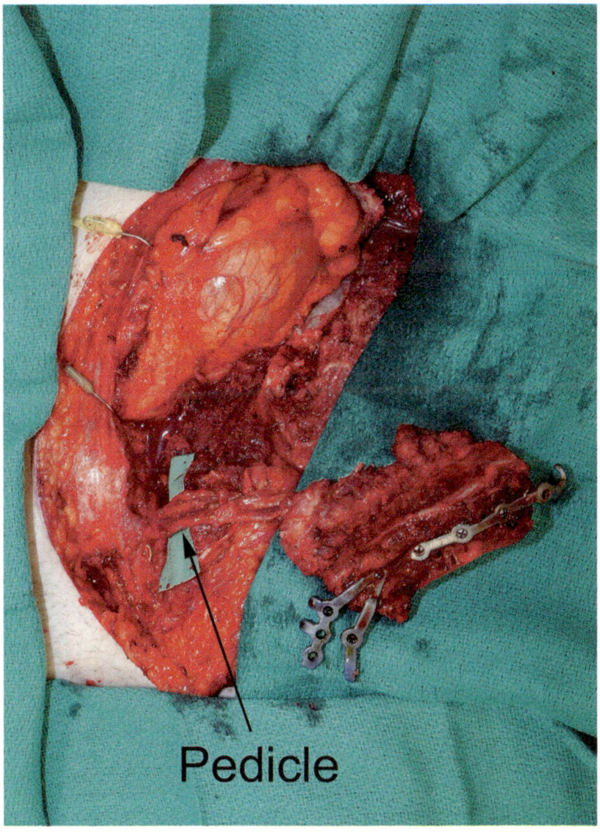

Fig. 8.8 Fully dissected iliac crest osseous free flap. A 3D printed titanium plate has been fixated to the bone. The anterior (medial) iliac crest flap will be fixated to the ramus of the mandible and the posterior (lateral) iliac crest will be fixated to the parasymphysis of the mandible

anteromedial thigh (AMT) cutaneous perforator free flap and a vastus lateralis muscle free flap were harvested from the right thigh (Fig. 8.9). The AMT was selected over an anterolateral thigh (ALT) free flap because of the presence of a much larger perforator supplying the flap. A custom 3D printed plate was used for rigid fixation to the mandibular remnants and microvascular anastomoses were performed to branches of the left external carotid artery and left facial vein (Fig. 8.10). The completed reconstruction is shown in Fig. 8.11.

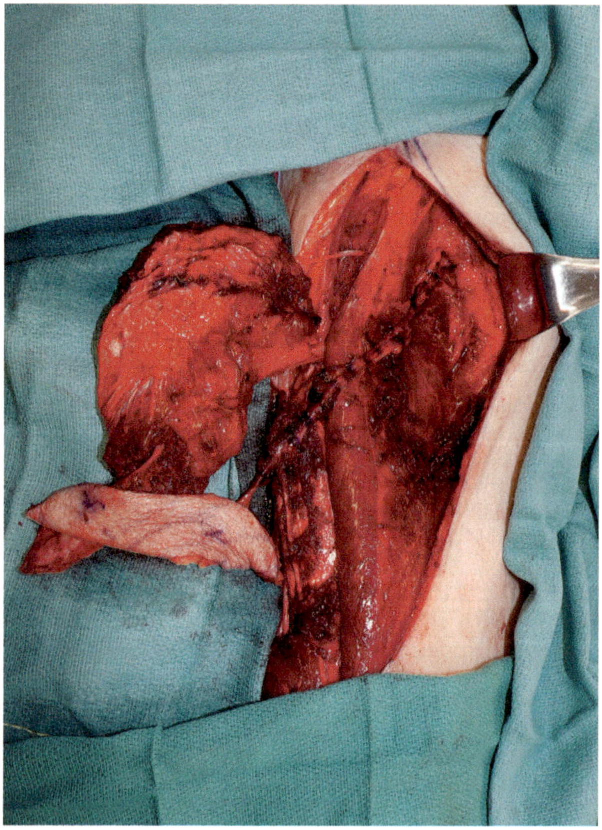

Fig. 8.9 Due to excessive soft tissue bulk, the skin over the iliac crest was not used for intraoral soft tissue reconstruction. Instead, an anteromedial thigh (AMT) cutaneous perforator free flap with a chimeric vastus lateralis muscle flap was harvested for intraoral and external neck reconstruction, respectively

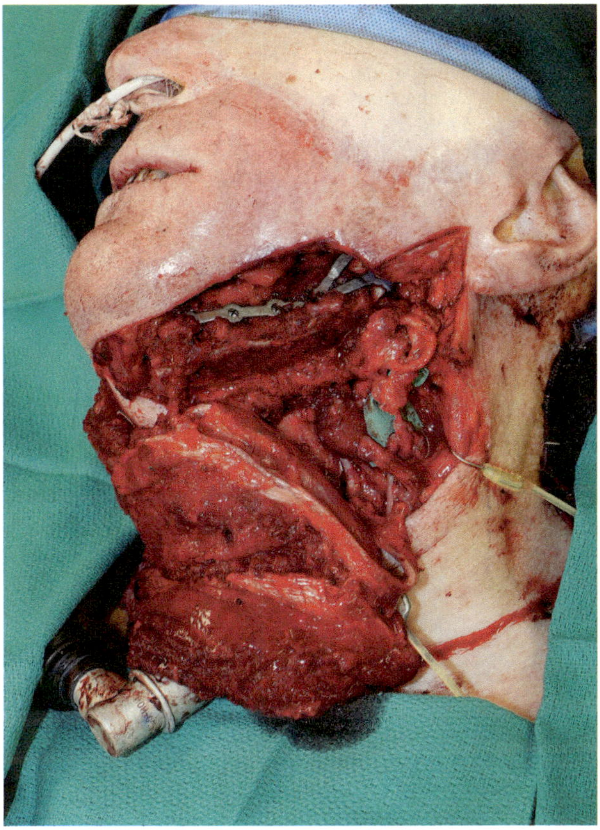

Fig. 8.10 Rigid fixation of the iliac crest bone free flap to the mandibular remnants as well as inset of the AMT cutaneous perforator free flap and anastomosis to branches of the left external carotid artery and facial vein

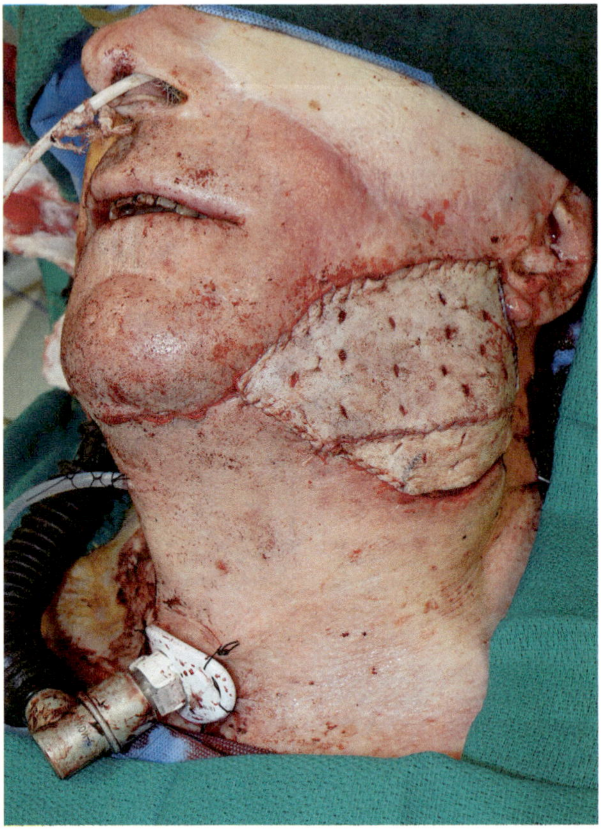

Fig. 8.11 Completed reconstruction with the vastus lateralis muscle flap covered by a full-thickness skin graft used to reconstruct the external neck

Summary Section

- The DCIA flap provides excellent quality and quantity of vascularized bone along with muscle and/or skin components, establishing it as an excellent alternative for patients who are not candidates for a free fibula flap.
- Modifications from the traditional iliac crest flap design have resulted in a flap that can be harvested without the internal oblique muscle solely based on a skin perforator which allows for improved skin paddle mobility and decreased bulk.
- The DCIA flap is an excellent option for both mandibular and maxillary reconstruction with its natural contour and robust bone stock allowing for full dental rehabilitation.
- While the vascular pedicle of the deep circumflex iliac artery and vein is relatively large in caliber and reliable in its anatomy, musculocutaneous perforators to support a skin paddle can be variable in number and location.
- Meticulous donor site closure is important to minimize donor site morbidity, particularly the formation of abdominal hernia.

References

1. Taylor GI, Townsend P, Corlett R. Superiority of the deep circumflex iliac vessels as the supply for free groin flaps: clinical work. Plast Reconstr Surg. 1979;64:745–59.
2. Kimata Y, Uchiyama K, Sakuraba M, et al. Deep circumflex iliac perforator flap with iliac crest for mandibular reconstruction. Br J Plast Surg. 2001;54:487–90.
3. Safak T, Klebuck MJA, Mavili E, Shenaq S. A new design of the iliac crest microsurgical free flap without including the "obligatory" muscle cuff. Plast Reconstr Surg. 1997;100:1703–9.
4. Shenaq SM, Klebuc MJ. Refinements in the iliac crest microsurgical free flap for oromandibular reconstruction. Microsurgery. 1994;15:825–30.
5. David DJ, Tan E, Katsaros J, Sheen R. Mandibular reconstruction with vascularized iliac crest: a 10-year experience. Plast Reconstr Surg. 1998;82:792–801.
6. Brown JS, Jones DC, Summerwill A, et al. Vascularized iliac crest with internal oblique muscle for immediate reconstruction after maxillectomy. Br J Oral Maxillofac Surg. 2002;40:183–90.
7. Delimar D, Bohacek I, Pecina M, Bicanic G. Acetabular roof reconstruction with pedicled iliac graft: ten years later. Int Orthop. 2014;38(1):199–201.
8. Zheng L, Wu W, Shi Y, Zhang J. Mandibular reconstruction with a deep circumflex iliac artery flap using computer-assisted and intraoral anastomosis techniques. J Oral Maxillofac Surg. 2019;77(12):2567–72.
9. Kim HS, Kim BC, Kim HJ, Kim HJ. Anatomical basis of the deep circumflex iliac artery flap. J Craniofac Surg. 2013 Mar;24(2):605–9.
10. Ramamastry SS, Granick MS, Futrell JW. Clinical anatomy of the internal oblique muscle. J Reconstr Microsurg. 1986;2:117–22.
11. Ting JW, Rozen WM, Grinsell D, Stella DL, Ashton MW. The in vivo anatomy of the deep circumflex iliac artery perforators: defining the role for the DCIA perforator flap. Microsurgery. 2009;29(4):326–9.
12. Bergeron L, Tang M, Morris SF. The anatomical basis of the deep circumflex iliac artery perforator flap with iliac crest. Plast Reconstr Surg. 2007;120:252–8.
13. Chandra SR, Morlandt A, Ying Y, Rana M, Acero J, Parmar S. Deep circumflex iliac artery-based composite flap or vascularized iliac crest flap. Atlas Oral Maxillofac Surg Clin North Am. 2023;31(2):113–20.

Chapter 9
Calvarial Bone Flaps

Maureen Beederman and Lawrence J. Gottlieb

Background

Cranioplasty with vascularized bone was first described in the German literature by Muller and then modified by Koenig in 1890 [1, 2]. These "osteoplastic flaps" transferred outer-table calvarial bone, attached to the pericranium and skin, to repair adjacent cranial defects with vascularized bone. During the same era, Wagner developed the osteoplastic craniotomy procedure elevating a full-thickness bone flap attached to the pericranium and skin to provide exposure to the brain for evacuation of hematomas or resection of tumors [3, 4]. Throughout the next century, there were a number of surgeons who developed modifications of calvarial bone grafts and osteoplastic flap cranioplasties and craniotomies [5–8]. In 1972, the first description of use of calvarial bone flaps for facial reconstruction was introduced by Conley, who detailed his use of multiple different pedicled composite flaps for head and neck reconstruction [9]. He noted that use of calvarial bone flaps had more robust blood supply and reduced donor site complications, when compared to other regional bone flaps harvested from the clavicle, rib, or scapula.

In 1984, McCarthy and Zide described a vascularized parietal bone flap based on the temporal vasculature emphasizing that the bone should be harvested cephalad to the temporal line [10]. They initially described using an outer-table calvarial bone flap carried on a pedicle of temporoparietal fascia, deep temporal fascia, periosteum, and temporalis muscle to reconstruct a malar deformity. A few months later, Cutting describes the blood supply to the parietal bone with the most significant finding that the superficial temporal artery sends perforator vessels down through the periosteum into the outer table of the parietal bone at a point

M. Beederman · L. J. Gottlieb (✉)
Section of Plastic and Reconstructive Surgery, The University of Chicago Medicine & Biological Sciences, Chicago, IL, USA
e-mail: lgottlie@bsd.uchicago.edu

J. P. Agarwal, D. W. Mathes (eds.), *Bone Flaps in Reconstructive Surgery*,
https://doi.org/10.1007/978-3-032-12540-8_9

approximately 1 to 2 cm beyond the temporal line [11]. Of note, although these authors initially included the temporalis muscle in their construct, they subsequently found that the temporalis muscle was not necessary to maintain vascularity of the parietal bone flap.

Over the next few decades there are a number of publications that describe pedicled calvarial flaps for midface reconstruction with pedicles based on the anterior deep and middle deep temporal arteries supplying the temporalis muscle [12–17], the posterior deep temporal artery (AKA middle temporal artery) supplying the subgaleal/innominate and deep temporal fascia [18, 19] and/or the superficial temporal artery supplying the temporoparietal (galeal) fascia [15, 20–25].

Indications

Calvarial bone flaps are predominantly used for reconstruction of defects of the calvarium, maxilla/midface, and mandible. It is a particularly useful option when one would otherwise use cranial bone graft but the wound bed is suboptimal because of scar, infection, or radiation. Maintaining the blood flow to the cranial bone flap will typically retain viable osteocytes, optimize bony union, and minimize resorption and infection. Calvarial bone flaps are also reliable alternative donor site options for patients who are unable or unwilling to use standard donor bone flaps such as the fibula, iliac crest, scapula, or radius. These flaps may be unavailable due to prior use or injury, occupational concerns, and other associated comorbidities, including peripheral vascular disease, lower extremity venous stasis, and lymphedema. The calvarial bone flap option is especially useful for osteocutaneous reconstruction in hair-bearing areas, such as the scalp, and mustache and beard distribution in male patients.

Hair-bearing soft tissue flaps to the face have a long history starting with a tubed pedicle flap by Gillies [26] and island flap based on the superficial temporal artery for reconstruction of an upper lip by Esser [27]. In 1974, Harii and colleagues were the first to report transferring a free hair-bearing scalp flap to the contralateral scalp with microvascular anastomoses in patients with burn alopecia so the hair would be oriented correctly [28]. Since then, there have been numerous reports of free and pedicled hair-bearing soft tissue flaps to other areas of the scalp or to the face in the literature [29–33]. In 1992, Gottlieb reconstructed an upper lip and anterior portion of maxilla, after wide excision on an indolent basal cell carcinoma, with a temporoparietal-osteo-fascio-cutaneous hair-bearing free flap containing the outer table of the parietal bone. This complex flap was transferred as a free flap for the ease of insetting and optimal orientation of not only the hair but all of the tissue

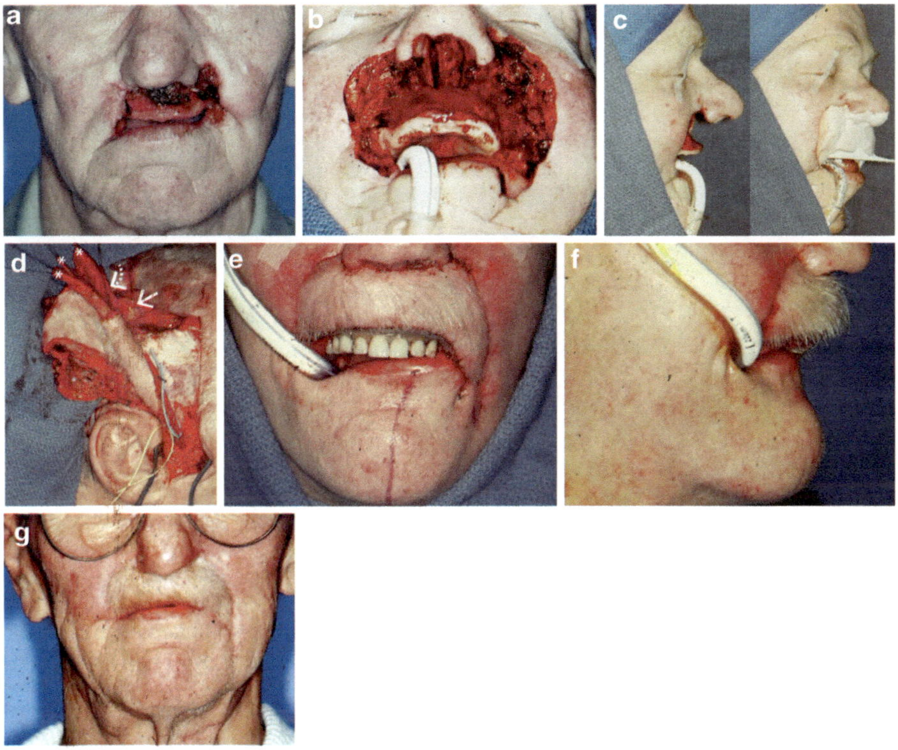

Fig. 9.1 Temporoparietal-osteo-fascio-cutaneous hair-bearing free flap containing the outer table of the parietal bone. (**a**) Indolent basal cell carcinoma of the upper lip in a 72-year-old male. (**b**) Defect after resection of upper lip (extending into cheeks), portion of lower lip, anterior surface of maxilla, nasal floor, and columella. (**c**) Lateral view demonstrating the volume of tissue missing. Alginate mold made for 3D perspective to aid in planning reconstruction. (**d**) Hair-bearing temporoparietal-osteo-fascial-cutaneous composite free flap based on the superficial temporal vessels. Vascularized outer table of cranium (straight arrow) to replace the anterior surface of the maxilla, various layers of temporoparietalis fascia (white asterisks) used to create the buccal sulcus and line the nasal floor, and subgaleal/innominate fascia (curved arrow) used to bring orbicularis muscle defect in attempt to recreate sphincter. Hair-bearing skin to recreate mustache. (**e**, **f**) At the completion of surgery, buccal lining created with a skin graft that was held in place with patient's denture, which was K-wired to hard palate. (**g**) Six months post-op of single-stage reconstruction with no revisions

components (Fig. 9.1). After collecting a series of hair-bearing flaps, this case was first presented in 2003 [34] and first published in 2012 [35]. Another patient in the series underwent a similar flap with full-thickness cranium and overlying skin to reconstruct an anterior mandible (Fig. 9.2).

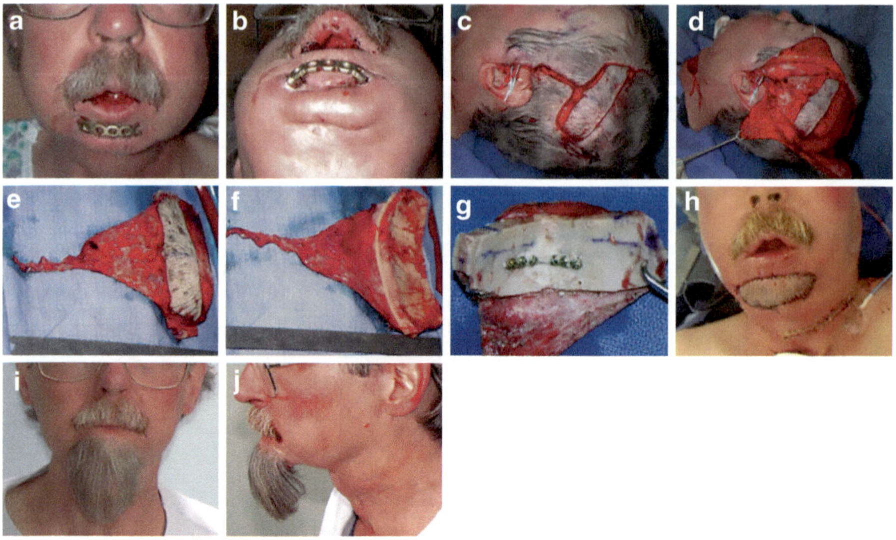

Fig. 9.2 Temporoparietal-osteo-fascio-cutaneous hair-bearing free flap containing full-thickness parietal bone. (**a**, **b**) A 50 y.o. male with plate extrusion one year following chemoradiation and mandibulectomy and reconstruction with RFFF and mandibular plate. Patient refused use of fibula due to occupation. (**c**) Skin paddle of hair-bearing osteocutaneous TPF. (**d**) Surrounding scalp elevated beneath galea as a rotation flap to close defect. (**e**) Pedicle divided and ready to be transferred to chin with bone and hair oriented correctly. (**f**) Undersurface of full-thickness calvarial osteocutaneous flap. (**g**) Osteotomy performed to obtain correct angle. (**h**) Skin inset. (**i**, **j**) Nine months post-op with excellent camouflage of flap

Anatomy Considerations

The soft tissue components of cranial bone flaps may include muscle, fascia, periosteum, subcutaneous tissue, and skin. The layers of the scalp in the temporoparietal region include the skin, subcutaneous tissue, temporoparietal fascia (TPF), loose areolar tissue (subgaleal/innominate fascia), temporalis fascia, temporalis muscle, pericranium, and bone. The TPF extends cranial as the galea aponeurotica and caudad as the superficial musculoaponeurotic system (SMAS).

The calvaria is the top part of the skull made up of the frontal, parietal, temporal, and occipital bones. The dominant blood supply to the calvaria is from the middle meningeal artery which is a branch of the maxillary artery that travels through the foramen spinosum to supply blood to the dura mater. It follows a fixed course as it embeds into a groove of the inner surface of the cranial bone. Since the middle meningeal artery is intimate with the dura and not easily accessed, it is not particularly useful as a vascular pedicle for a bone flap.

Although the blood supply to the calvarium is mostly from branches of the external carotid artery, the supraorbital and supratrochlear arteries (branches of the internal carotid system) provide a vascular supply to the outer cortex of the frontal bone.

Bone flaps based on these vessels have been used for frontal sinus obliteration and nasal/periorbital reconstruction [36, 37] (Fig. 9.3).

The anatomy of the scalp and cranium has been described in standard anatomic textbooks. Although most anatomists are in agreement with the description and terminology of the layers of the scalp in the frontal and occipital areas, there are significant disparate thoughts regarding the anatomic layers of the temporoparietal area, its blood supply, and its nomenclature. New excitement was generated in this topic with the search for calvarial flaps initiated by McCarthy's group in 1984 [11]. Since then, four major groups published on variations of anatomy and discussions of description (sometimes just semantics) and significance of various layers in the temporoparietal region of the scalp and its blood supply [15, 38–40]. Implications of how these layers may affect the transfer of vascularized bone flaps are most significant to this chapter. In 1986, Acland's group examined the surgical anatomy of the blood supply of the fascial layers of the temporoparietal region. The most significant new finding was that the middle temporal artery (some call the deep posterior temporal artery) was the primary blood supply to the deep temporal fascia. Of significance, primarily for pedicled flaps, the middle temporal artery is a branch off of the proximal portion of the STA [38]. In the same year, Grotting's group studied and provided additional detail regarding the blood supply to the calvarium. They describe (or rename) a new layer that they called the innominate fascia that was deep to the temporoparietal (galeal) layer and superficial to the deep temporal fascia (overlying the temporalis muscle). They claimed that one only needed to include the innominate fascia and deep temporal fascia (aponeurosis) to maintain adequate blood supply for outer-table calvarial bone

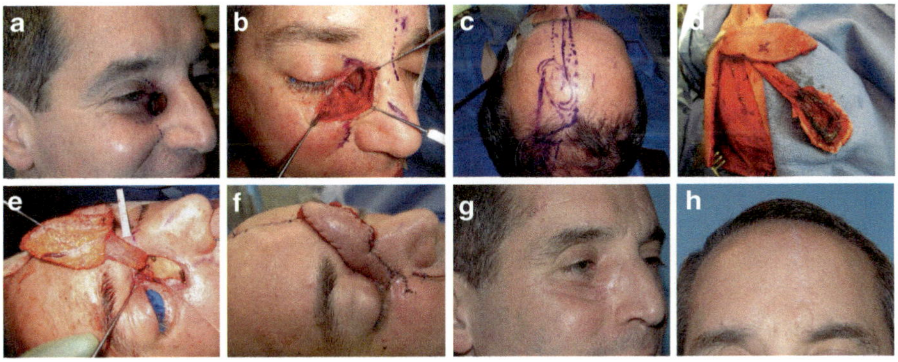

Fig. 9.3 Supratrochlear split calvarial osteo-myocutaneous paramedian forehead flap. (**a**) A 46 y.o. male with a history of sinonasal undifferentiated carcinoma initially treated with surgical resection and proton beam radiation and subsequently with conventional chemoradiation with a complex wound located next to patient's dominant eye. (**b**) Defining defect of mucosa, bone, and skin. (**c**) Flap design with a paramedian forehead flap with a galeal/periosteal extension of frontalis muscle carrying outer table harvested behind hairline. (**d**) Forehead skin and muscle separated with outer table of skull attached to muscle, galea, and pericranium (**e**) Frontalis muscle used for lining and cranial bone trimmed and rigidly fixed. (**f**) Skin inset. (**g**) One year post-op after division and insetting. (**h**) Forehead donor site

flaps [39]. In 1991 Tolhurst revisited the surgical anatomy of the scalp, attempted to "clean up" the nomenclature and described a new layer called the subgaleal layer which they state is a substantial, vascularized layer. This layer was similar to Casanova's innominate layer. They also believe that what others call subperiosteum layer is the true periosteal layer [40]. In 1995, Nakajima further investigated the vascular anatomy of the temporoparietal region providing a new understanding of the arterial vascular networks and their interconnections [15].

To summarize these anatomic findings, the STA supplies the skin and subcutaneous tissue superficial to it and the TPA and loose areola (subgaleal or innominate) fascia deep to it. As it extends beyond the temporal line over the parietal bone, it sends branches to pierce the innominate fascia and periosteum to penetrate the outer cortex of the parietal bone. The middle temporal artery (some call it the posterior deep temporal artery) which is a proximal branch of the STA, supplies the subgaleal/innominate fascia and deep temporal fascia lying on the temporalis muscle with a muscular branch going to the temporalis muscle. The temporalis muscle is primarily supplied by the anterior deep temporal and middle deep temporal arteries which take origin from the second portion of the internal maxillary artery. These vessels provide the blood supply to the outer cortex of the temporal bone. The blood supply to the parietal bone comes from three sources (in addition to the middle meningeal artery on the medial or cranial side of the bone), which are the blood vessels running in the temporalis muscle, the subgaleal/innominate (loose areola) fascia, and the temporoparietal fascia. These layers join at the level of the superior temporal line. As mentioned above, the STA pierces the innominate fascia and periosteum to penetrate the outer cortex of the parietal bone 1 to 2 cm cranial to this line [11, 15, 39, 40] (Fig. 9.4).

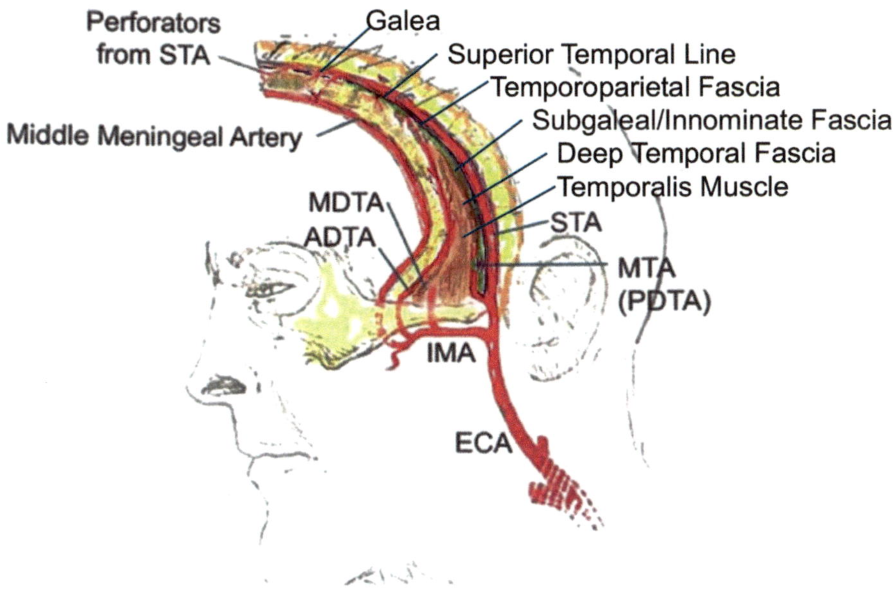

Fig. 9.4 Blood supply of temporoparietal area. The external carotid artery (ECA) give off the internal maxillary artery (IMA) and the superficial temporal artery (STA). The IMA gives off the anterior deep temporal artery (ADTA) and the middle deep temporal artery (MDTA) which lies below and provides blood supply to the temporalis muscle and also gives off the middle meningeal artery which is the source of most blood supply to the inner calvarial table. The STA gives off the posterior deep temporal artery (PDTA) also known as the middle temporal artery (MTA) which primarily provides blood flow to the deep temporal fascia with small branches to the temporal muscle. The STA sends branches to the calvarium 1–2 cm above the superior temporal line. (Modified from Clinics in Plastic Surgery Vol.14, No.1, 37–47. January 1987)

Dissection Considerations

Dissection of the temporoparietal region is individualized depending on components of the flap needed and which blood supply to the calvarium is used. These bone flaps may be harvested either as a full-thickness or split calvarial osteo-fascio or osteo-fascio-cutaneous flaps, depending on the amount and thickness of bone stock needed for the defect and whether or not skin is required.

To transfer temporal bone, the attached temporalis muscle, supplied by the anterior deep and/or middle deep temporal arteries, must be included. Although the temporalis muscle has been shown to be able to keep parietal bone flaps vascularized [13–17], it is not necessary for maintenance of the circulation of parietal calvarial bone flaps. Outer-table parietal calvarial flaps may be transferred on the deep temporal and subgaleal/innominate fascia primarily supplied by the proximal STA and its middle temporal branch. To optimize the blood supply of full-thickness parietal calvarial bone flaps, the pedicle should include the TPF with the superficial temporal vessels.

Those patients in whom the components of the flap are only bone with attached pericranium, fascia and blood vessels usually undergo a hemi- or bicoronal incision (Fig. 9.5). Dissection typically begins in the preauricular area where, in the vicinity of the zygomatic arch, the TPF attachment to the subcutaneous tissue is relatively loose compared to the intimate relationship of TPF to subcutaneous tissue more cranial. The superficial temporal artery and vein are identified (and isolated, skeletonized, and looped in free flap cases). Of note, the superficial temporal vein may not be immediately adjacent to the artery and may found up to 2–3 cm away. It usually has an external diameter of 2.1–3.3 mm and is located anterior to the artery. As one dissects inferiorly, the vessels get closer to each other. Ideally, the parietal calvarial bone donor site is selected 1 to 2 cm superior to the temporal line, away from the superior sagittal sinus and preferably placed posterior to (behind) the hairline, if possible. As dissection progresses cranially toward the area of proposed calvarial bone flap harvest, sharp dissection in a plane just deep to the hair follicles to separate the subcutaneous tissue from the underlying TPF is required. Care should be taken to minimize damage to vessels on one side and hair follicles on the other.

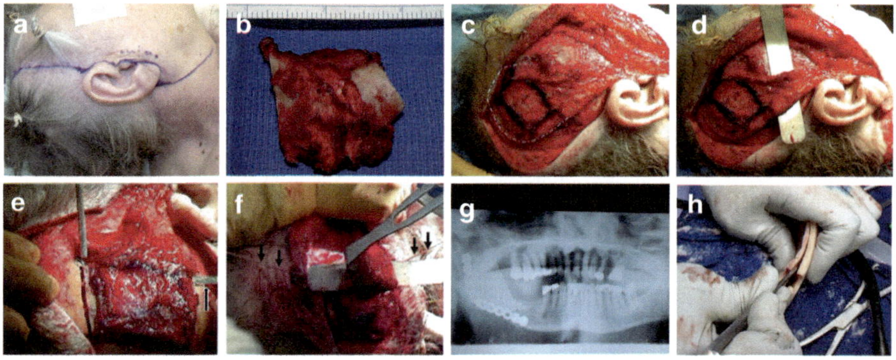

Fig. 9.5 Pedicled full-thickness osteofascial parietal bone flap. (**a**) Preauricular incision with cranial extension to harvest full-thickness parietal bone flap based on TPF supplied by the STA. Neck incision for tumor extirpation and neck dissection in an 81-year-old female with obesity and diabetes with an ameloblastoma carcinoma of the right mandible angle. On physical exam, her legs were edematous with evidence of venous stasis, precluding the use of her fibula for reconstruction. (**b**) Excised specimen. (**c**) Area of bone required is marked on the anticipated donor site. The TPF is then incised through pericranium (dashed line) about 1cm beyond the template border on all sides except the inferior margin which is left intact as it is attached to the vascular pedicle. (**d**) Malleable retractor is placed beneath the TPF and attached subgaleal/innominate fascia pedicle after it was elevated off the deep temporal fascia. (**e**) After bone was cut with a side-cutting guarded craniotome connecting the holes superiorly, anteriorly, and posteriorly, a flexible metal guide (arrow) is placed between the inferior holes to avoid injuring the dura as Gigli saw is passed. (**f**) TPF pedicle is elevated with an army-navy retractor and protected by a malleable retractor as the Gigli saw (black arrows) completes the inferior osteotomy. (**g**) Post-op Panorex. (**h**) Splitting bone graft to reconstruct donor site

Once the size of the recipient defect is known, a template is designed, placed, and then marked on the anticipated donor site taking into account the length of the pedicle as well as the pivot point for pedicled flaps. The temporoparietal fascia (TPF) (galea) is then incised through the pericranium about 1 cm beyond the template border on all sides except the inferior margin which is left intact as it is attached to the vascular pedicle (Fig. 9.5c). The TPF and attached subgaleal/innominate fascia pedicle is then elevated off of the deep temporal fascia from the preauricular area to the inferior margin of the template where it attaches to the bone (Fig. 9.5d). The remainder of the bicoronal incision (away from the bone flap) is raised in the supraperiosteal or subgaleal plane.

To harvest a split thickness calvarial flap, a trough is made around the area marked out for the bone flap, and then with an osteotome or Gigli saw, the outer table is separated from the inner table through the diploe. Usually the inferior bone cut, the portion under the pedicle, can be either manually osteotomized or sometimes a Gigli saw is needed to complete that osteotomy being careful to not injure the overlying pedicle. If a full-thickness cranial bone flap is planned, then neurosurgery is consulted to elevate a full-thickness calvarial bone flap off the dura. Typically 3 or 4 burr holes are created around the bone flap. The dura is dissected from the bone between the burr holes and the bone is then cut with a side-cutting guarded craniotome connecting the holes superiorly, anteriorly, and posteriorly. A Gigli saw is then used to complete the last osteotomy (inferior to attachment of the pedicle). Typically the Gigli saw is attached to a flexible metal guide to avoid injuring the dura (Fig. 9.5e–f). In both split and full-thickness bone flap harvest, small holes are drilled along the edge of the bone so the pericranial tissue can be secured to it with absorbable sutures to avoid inadvertent shearing and disruption of the fine network of vessels connecting the pedicle to the bone. The pedicle of the flap is then dissected proximally until sufficient pedicle length is achieved for placement of the flap in the recipient site (Fig. 9.6). Some flaps are difficult to orient correctly or are too bulky to be passed through soft tissue tunnels while attached to its pedicle. In those cases, it is usually best to transfer it as a free flap, dividing the artery and vein and then performing microvascular anastomoses to a convenient recipient vessel.

If a full-thickness bone flap is used, the calvarial donor site is resurfaced by a separate split calvarial bone graft harvested from another site on the skull or alloplastic material may be employed (Fig. 9.5h).

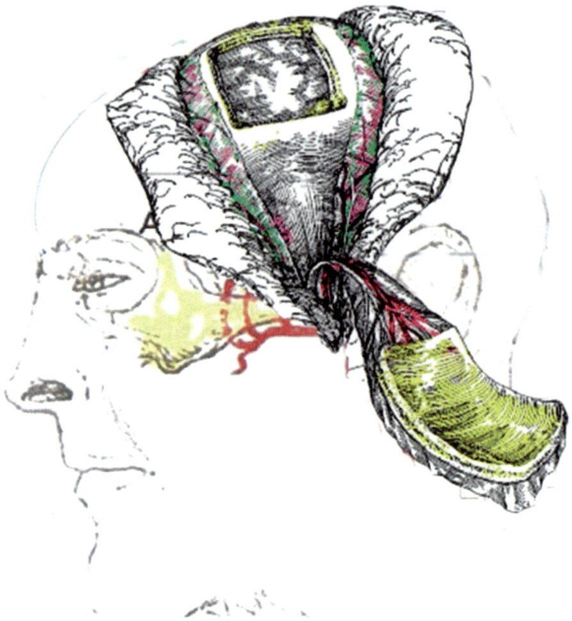

Fig. 9.6 Temporoparietal-osseous flap ready for transfer as a pedicled or free flap. (Modified from page 639 in Serafin [41])

Summary

While initially described more than a century ago and popularized in the 1970s and 1980s, calvarial bone flaps have largely gone out of favor. Due to the success of distraction osteogenesis techniques for many congenital craniofacial deformities and the increasing reliability and perhaps familiarity with microsurgical transfer of distant tissue (vascularized fibula, iliac crest, and scapula) for acquired defects from trauma or oncologic resection, the use of cranial bone flaps have more recently taken a back seat and is at risk of becoming a lost art. However, we believe this flap should remain an important part of the plastic surgeon's armamentarium for reconstruction of calvarial, midface, and mandibular defects. The use of vascularized calvarial bone often allows for improved contouring, a donor site with minimal discomfort and complications, and the unique ability to reconstruct the hair-bearing regions of the scalp, mustache, and beard distributions with unparalleled results.

References

1. Beck C. Cranioplastic operations. JAMA. 1894;23:803.
2. Flanigan P, Kshettry VR, Benzel EC. World War II, tantalum, and the evolution of modern cranioplasty technique. Neurosurg Focus. 2014:36. https://doi.org/10.3171/2014.2.FOCUS13552.

3. Goodrich JT. How to get in and out of the skull: from tumi to "hammer and chisel" to the Gigli saw and the osteoplastic flap. Neurosurg Focus. 2014;36(4):E6. https://doi.org/10.3171/2014.2.FOCUS13543.
4. Buchfelder M, Ljunggren B. Wilhelm Wagner (1848-1900): Part 2: The Osteoplastic Flap. Surg Neurol. 1988;30:428–33.
5. Watson Jones R. The repair of the skull defects by a new pedicle bone graft operation. Br Med J. 1933;I:780.
6. González-Darder JM, Capilla-Guasch P. The temporary resection of the cranial vault by Wilhelm Wagner (1848–1900) instead of trepanation: the cornerstone of the modern craniotomy. J Neurosurg. 2023;139:573–8.
7. Stricker M, Montaut J, Hepner H, Flot F. Les ostéotomies du crâne et de la face [Osteotomy of the skull and face]. Ann Chir Plast. 1972;17(4):233–44. French PMID: 4642545.
8. Vandervord JG, Watson JD, Teasdale GM. Forehead reconstruction using a bi-pedicled bone flap. Br J Plast Surg. 1982;35:75–9.
9. Conley J. Use of composite flaps containing bone for major repairs in the head and neck. Plast Reconstr Surg. 1972;49(5):522–6.
10. McCarthy JG, Zide BM. The spectrum of calvarial bone grafting: introduction of the vascularized calvarial bone flap. Plast Reconstr Surg. 1984;74(1):10–8.
11. Cutting CB, McCarthy JG, Berenstein A. Blood supply of the upper craniofacial skeleton: the search for composite calvarial bone flaps. Plast Reconstr Surg. 1984;74(5):603–10.
12. Bite U, Jackson IT, Wahner HW, et al. Vascularized skull bone grafts in craniofacial surgery. Ann Plast Surg. 1987;19:3.
13. Holtje WJ, Schwipper V. The temporalis osteomyoperiosteal flap: its blood supply and use for reconstruction of the maxilla. Eur J Plast Surg. 1989;12:245–54.
14. Gratz KW, Sailer HF, Haers PE, Oechslin CK. Mandibular reconstruction with full thickness calvarial bone and temporal muscle flap. Br J Oral Maxillofac Surg. 1996;34:379–85.
15. Nakajima H, Imanishi N, Minabe T. The arterial anatomy of the temporal region and the vascular basis of various temporal flaps. Br J Plast Surg. 1995;48(7):439–50.
16. Antonyshyn O, Colcleugh RG, Hurst LN, et al. The temporalis myoosseous flap: an experimental study. Plast Reconstr Surg. 1986;77:406.
17. Van der Meulen JC, Hauben DJ, Vaanderager JM, Birgenhager- Frenkel DH. The use of a temporal osteoperiosteal flap for the reconstruction of malar hypoplasia in Treacher Collins syndrome. Plast Reconstr Surg. 1984;74:687–93.
18. Psillakis JM, Grotting JC, Casanova R, et al. Vascularized outer-table calvarial bone flaps. Plast Reconstr Surg. 1986;78:308.
19. Grotting JC, Psillakis, Casanova R, Vasconez LO. Craniofacial reconstruction after tumor resections using vascularized outer table calvarial bone flaps. Am J Surg. 1998;152:438–41.
20. Munoz FI, Juncosa AM, Carillo FO. Vascularized Parietal Bone Flaps. A new dimension in Mandibular reconstruction. J Cranio-Max-Fac Surg. 1990;18:158–63.
21. Parhiscar A, Har-El G, Turk JB, Abramson DL. Temporoparietal osteofascial flap for head and neck reconstruction. J Oral Maxillofac Surg. 2002;60(6):619–22. https://doi.org/10.1053/joms.2002.33104. PMID: 12022094.
22. Davison SP, Mesbahi AN, Clemens MW, Picken CA. Vascularized calvarial bone flaps and midface reconstruction. Plast Reconstr Surg. 2008;122(1):10e.
23. Bilen BT, Kılınc H, Arslan A, et al. Reconstruction of orbital floor and maxilla with divided vascularised calvarial bone flap in one session. J Plast Reconstr Aesthet Surg. 2006;59:1305e11.
24. Kamljl T, Fujikawa M, Honda T, Hlgasa H, Sekiguchl J, Ohmori K. Restoration of the mandible by full-thickness calvarial bone flap. Ann Plast Surg. 1992;29:438–43.
25. Choung PH, Nam IW, Kin KS. Vascularized cranial bone grafts. J Cranio-Max-Fac Surg. 1991;19:235–42.
26. Gillies HS. Injuries to Upper lip. Ch 111, pg 39 Plastic Surgery of the face. Oxford University Press; 1920.
27. Esser JFS. Preservation of innervation and circulation supply in plastic restoration of upper lip. Ann Surg. 1934;99(1):101–11.

28. Harii K, Ohmori K, Ohmori S, Harii KMD. Hair transplantation with free scalp flaps. Plastic Reconstr Surg. 1974;53(4):410–3.
29. Ohmori K. Free Scalp Flap. Plastic Reconstr Surg. 1980;65(I):42–9.
30. Juri J, Juri C. Two new methods of treating baldness: temporo-parieto-occipito-parietal pedicled flap and temporo-parieto-occipital free flap. Ann Plast Surg. 1981;6:38.
31. Buncke HJ, Hoffman WY, Alpert BS, Gordon L, Stefani AE. Microvascular transplantation of two free scalp flaps between identical twins. Plast Reconstr Surg. 1982;70:605.
32. Walton RL, Bunkis J. A free occipital hair-bearing flap for reconstruction of the upper lip. Br J Plastic Surg. 1983;36:168–I70.
33. Ridgway EB, Pribaz JJ. The reconstruction of male hair-bearing facial regions. Plast Reconstr Surg. 2011;127(1):131–41.
34. Gottlieb LJ, Hornik B. Camouflage Free Flaps. The aesthetic facial reconstruction in adults and children meeting. Arizona: Plastic Surgery Educational Foundation; 2003.
35. Gottlieb LJ, Agarwal S. Autologous alternatives to face transplant. J Reconstr Microsurg. 2012;28:49–61.
36. McCarthy JG, Cutting CB, Shaw WW. Clin Plast Surg. 1987;14(1):37–47.
37. Ooi ASH, Gottlieb LJ. Pedicled flaps in head and neck reconstruction. In: Matthew Hanasono M, Samir Mardini S, Moran S, editors. Problem-solving in reconstructive surgery. CRC Press; 2019.
38. Abul-Hassan HS, von Drasek Ascher G, Acland RD. Surgical anatomy and blood supply of the fascial layers of- the temporal region. Plast Reconstr Surg. 1986;77:17–24.
39. Casanova R, Cavalcante D, Grotting JC, Vasconez LO, Psillakis JM. Anatomic basis for vascularized outer-table calvarial bone flaps. Plast Reconstr Surg. 1986;78(3):300–8. https://doi.org/10.1097/00006534-198609000-00004. PMID: 3737754.
40. Tolhurst DE, Carstens MH, Greco RJ, Hurwitz DJ. The surgical anatomy of the scalp. Plast Reconstr Surg. 1991;87:603–12.
41. Serafin DG. Atlas on microsurgical composite tissue transplantation. Chapter 59. In: The Calvarial Osseous Flap. Saunders; 1996.

Chapter 10
Spino-Plastics: Revolutionizing Spinal Reconstruction with Vascularized Bone Grafts

Casey Martinez, Sebastian Winocour, and Edward Reece

Introduction: Setting the Stage for Innovation

Overview of Spinal Surgery

The aging global population has shed light on spinal pathology, calling into question the current treatment options as the burden of disease and concomitant comorbidities continues to rise [1, 2]. Rising healthcare costs associated with spinal fusion are not only due to the rise in incidence of spine issues, but are in part due to the unfortunately high reoperation rate status post failed fusion with traditional use of nonvascularized bone grafts (N-VBGs) and allografts [2]. The field of spino-plastics is tasked with addressing this pressing problem. Patients who did not have satisfactory outcomes of spinal instrumentation and fusion, which led to pseudoarthrosis, are candidates for vascularized bone grafts (VBGs). VBGs, which can be taken from the iliac crest (IC-VBG), rib (R-VBG), spinous process (SP-VBG), scapula (S-VBG), occiput (O-VBG), and clavicle (C-VBG) can be utilized in adjunct to spinal instrumentation to augment healing and fusion capabilities (Table 10.1) [3]. For the past two decades, plastic surgeons have taken on a more robust role as spine surgeons, joining orthopedic surgeons and neurosurgeons. Options for reconstruction have grown to include VBGs among other complex wound closures to improve spinal fusion rates while minimizing patient morbidity [4].

C. Martinez
Alix School of Medicine, Mayo Clinic, Phoenix, AZ, USA

S. Winocour
Department of Plastic Surgery, Baylor College of Medicine, Houston, TX, USA

E. Reece (✉)
Division of Plastic Surgery, Mayo Clinic, Phoenix, AZ, USA
e-mail: edwardreece@edwardreece.com

J. P. Agarwal, D. W. Mathes (eds.), *Bone Flaps in Reconstructive Surgery*,
https://doi.org/10.1007/978-3-032-12540-8_10

Table 10.1 Each type of VBG with corresponding arc of rotation, vascular pedicle, and other considerations

VBG type	Arc of rotation	Pedicle	Contribution to Sharpey's fibers	Preservation of important structures	Other notes
IC-VBG	T12–sacrum	Quadratus lumborum	Multifactorial	Cluneal nerve	First line for VBG of distal thoracic and lumbar spine
O-VBG	C1–T1	Splenius capitis; semispinalis capitis	Deep cervical artery	Foramen magnum	Mathes-Nahai type 2
S-VBG	Occiput–T8	Rhomboid minor; trapezius	Multifactorial	Descending branch of the transverse cervical artery	
R-VBG	C6–L5 (for eighth rib)	Subcostals	Subcostal artery	Intercostal nerve; lung pleura	Rib curvature and location taken into consideration; ensure no pneumothorax
SP-VBG	Thoracolumbar spine	Paraspinals	Paraspinal perforators		Ensure adequate fixation and surgical planning to avoid injury to harvest site at time of instrumentation/ fixation
C-VBG	C2–T2	Clavicular head of the SCM	Branches of occipital and superior thyroid arteries	Anterior cervical neurovasculature	Anterior cervicothoracic spinal defects

Understanding Vertebral Body Defects

There are a wide range of vertebral body defects that stem from congenital deformities to cancer, trauma, infection, and neurodegenerative etiologies [5, 6]. Treatment options are highly specific to location, presentation, severity of disease, appearance on imaging, and patient status, among other characteristics. When conservative treatments are no longer an option, surgical intervention may be explored. First, minimally invasive approaches including vertebral augmentation procedures might be considered if there is no severe deformity, instability, cord compression, cement allergy, chronic fracture or vertebra planae, or any other contraindication [7, 8]. The more complex the case, the more likely the probability that procedures such as balloon kyphoplasty or vertebroplasty might result in poor outcomes, with complications including cement extravasation and compression fracture at adjacent vertebral levels [7, 9]. When clinical picture or severity at presentation favor an open surgical approach, spinal instrumentation and fusion offers a more substantive repair with potential for nerve decompression, with restoration of segment length, curvature, and stabilization [10, 11]. Annual rates of spinal fusion more than doubled from 1998 to 2008, and the most common indication has been degenerative conditions [2, 12].

There is a significant amount of ambiguity within the literature behind rates of complication and failure for arthrodesis [13, 14]. Pseudoarthrosis is a very serious potential complication that can be quite challenging to address, with some sources citing pseudoarthrosis rates as rare as less than 2%, while others cite greater than 60% occurrence [14–16]. In the case of spinal metastasis, for example, rates of surgical intervention in the pediatric population have increased, and yet, there has been little improvement in outcomes such as complication or mortality rates [17]. One possible explanation for this lack of clarity is patient cohort selection, as there are several variables that have a profound effect on outcomes, including surgical approach, internal fixation technique, site preparation, degree of deformity, length and location of affected segment, and patient factors like age, smoking status, etc. [15, 16, 18, 19] Pseudoarthrosis is just one of the many possible complications of spinal fusion. The procedure may not resolve the inciting neck or back pain, but instead may even worsen this discomfort, causing radiculopathy, myelopathy, or neurological deficits [15, 20].

The Evolution of VBGs

A Historical Perspective

The first described vascularized bone transfer was in 1908; however, bony reconstruction has been attempted for thousands of years with a slow evolution towards vascular preservation [21, 22]. It was not until the 1990s that VBG's efficacy was proven to be superior to N-VBGs, when IC-VBGs were shown to have double the innate strength compared to their nonvascularized counterparts [23]. By definition, VBGs are a flap, as they carry their blood supply to the donor site, despite not always having a true named blood supply. While there are named vessels located within the muscle pedicle of various VBG types, the primary vasculature supply is directly from Sharpey's fibers, which are found in the periosteum and microvasculature of Haversian canals/musculature [24]. As such, there is a need to incorporate VBGs into the traditional reconstructive ladder or Gottlieb and Krieger's elevator: direct closure, skin graft, local flap, distant flap, tissue expansion, and microvascular [25]. One journal article proposed a new bony reconstruction algorithm with the following rungs: allograft, bony substitute, autograft, nonvascularized bone graft (N-VBG), vascularized bone graft (VBG), pedicled vascularized bone flap, and finally free bone flap [24].

Successful bone replacement was first achieved in the nineteenth century, with research subsequently paving the way for biological products, including platelet-rich plasma, hydroxyapatite, demineralized bone matrix, and various growth factor mixtures, as well as synthetic products, inclusive of polymers, ceramics composed of calcium with other supplemental elements, bioactive glass, and so much more [26]. Some smaller bony defects may not necessitate vascular supply to maintain structural integrity in the postoperative period, yet risk of failure does correlate with defect size. Despite technologic and scientific advancement, there remains much to be accomplished to achieve an adequate bony substitute with porous structure supporting vascularization in the setting of large bony defects [26]. There are several clinical scenarios where good patient outcomes and sufficient healing requires further support through a vascular supply that may not be achieved without vascularized bone grafting.

Mechanisms of Success

There are many biological underpinnings and therapeutic mechanisms allowing VBG to augment spinal fusion. Firstly, VBGs inherently maintain osteogenic, osteoinductive, and osteoconductive properties that promote direct healing instead of creeping substitution of N-VBGs [24, 27–31]. While providing robust blood supply, the VBG's muscular pedicle closes dead space, a factor that has been proven to reduce wound complications and reoperation rates [32]. Autografting carries much lower risk of rejection or allergic reaction as compared to allografting or introducing foreign materials and biologic substitutes. Because VBGs function similarly to local flaps, there is no microsurgical anastomosis or distant donor site morbidity as is found in free flaps [27–30]. With a more simple surgical procedure, there is a decrease in operative time, potential damage to donor site functioning, patient recovery time, and overall healthcare expenditure [33, 34].

Clinical Indications

The versatility and efficacy of VBGs promotes utilization of this invaluable tool in cases of complex spinal reconstruction. Complexity substantially increases in conditions that inhibit healthy vascularization, nutrient supply, and general viability of the recipient tissue bed, such as in cases of extensive traumatic injuries, large oncologic resections, osteomyelitis, or deep infection resulting in necrosis, radiation, significant kyphoscoliosis, osteopenia/osteoporosis, neuromuscular disease, immunosuppression, prior surgery to the affected area, or severe native tissue anomalies/malformations [24, 27–31, 35, 36]. At this point in time, it is more common to utilize VBGs in the setting of salvage reconstructive procedures, as compared to primary reconstruction. The vascularity provides additional biologic advantage, especially in cases of prior failed reconstruction and, therefore, further justification for a VBG. Yet there is an opportunity to use VBGs primarily in cases of high-risk patient populations. Unfortunately, identification of patients at risk for nonunion or malunion prior to initial fusion surgery is not always straightforward. There is a poor understanding behind the multifactorial basis for suboptimal fusion rates that result in decline in patient functional status and quality of life metrics [37].

Anatomic Choices and Technique in VBG

The Iliac Crest

The gold standard treatment for failed arthrodesis has been a nonvascularized iliac crest bone graft for augmentation of repeat arthrodesis; however, there have been many studies showing successful, and potentially superior, osteogenicity and fusion with utilization of the IC-VBG [38–43]. This is a great option for distal thoracic and lumbar spine defects, with feasibility to reach from T12 to the sacrum. Following the instrumentation and fixation, a ninety-degree unilateral incision is made from midline to the posterior superior iliac spine. Dissection and cauterization from skin to the iliac crest is performed subperiosteally to preserve the cluneal nerve and vascular supply to the quadratus lumborum muscular pedicle. Tricortical cancellous bone is excised by an ultrasonic bone scalpel or osteotome to cover the spinal defect, with a maximum recommended length of 12 cm. The multifidus and longissimus musculature is raised by blunt dissection and the released IC-VBG is tunneled submuscularly. The medullary portion of the VBG is then fixed to the decorticated spinal surface using plates and screws or titanium cables (Fig. 10.1). Placement is adjacent to the titanium instrumentation, as well as deep to the longissimus musculature.

The Occiput

O-VBGs are an excellent option for patients requiring strengthened fusion of the proximal spine, primarily C1 to T1 coverage and up to 5 cm in length [27, 44–46]. The deep cervical artery supplies the splenius capitis or semispinalis capitis muscular pedicle with very safe inferior rotation capability, due to the Mathes-Nahai type 2 classification. For this procedure, the patient is in the prone position and the spinal surgeon stabilizes the spine with adequate instrumentation. Then, a vertical incision is made from the greater occipital protuberance to the most distal aspect of the spinal defect. The surgeon must dissect the fascial plane between the semispinalis capitis and trapezius muscles. The median nuchal line and the foramen magnum are the anatomical borders, with the superior and lateral borders dictated by the size of the spinal defect. Subperiosteal dissection preserves graft vascularity

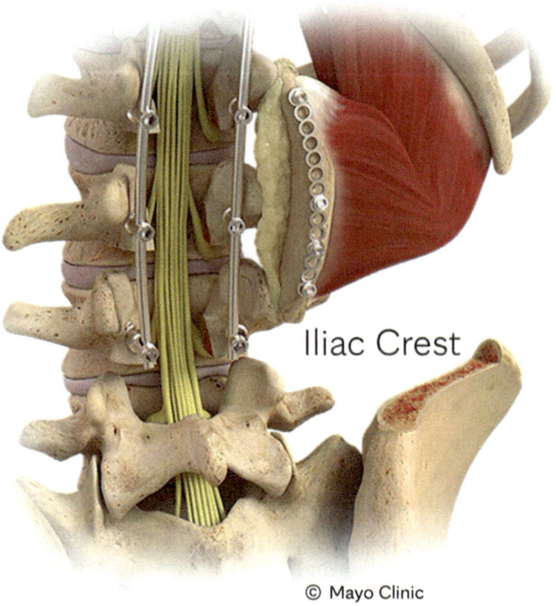

Fig. 10.1 IC-VBG pedicled on quadratus lumborum musculature, reproduced with permission from the Mayo Clinic

and an osteotome can be used to excise the O-VBG. The pedicle is then rotated to approximate the decorticated spinal edge with the leading edge of the graft (Fig. 10.2). Prior to closure, the trapezius musculature is advanced, overlying the affected area to fill the dead space.

The Scapula

In addition to O-VBGs, the S-VBG may provide great coverage for cervical spine defects, and the S-VBG arc of rotation is from the occiput to T8 level, with a maximum of 8–10 cm in length [20, 29, 47–49]. There is a heightened degree of importance to ensure adequate stabilization of the cervical spine due to the naturally greater degree of mobility of this proximal spine and close proximity to vital neurovascular structures [20]. After the spinal instrumentation is performed, from midline to the medial scapular border, an incision is made, with the length determined by size and level of the bony graft targeted for harvest. Careful dissection is performed beyond the paraspinal muscles, with special attention to avoid the transverse cervical artery along the medial scapula. The defect size is taken into account, and after subperiosteal dissection, keeping Sharpey's fibers to the trapezius and rhomboid muscles attached, an osteotome is used for the longitudinal excision of the scapula. The subscapularis is divided inferiorly to superiorly with termination before the descending branch of the transverse cervical artery. The S-VBG is next rotated on the trapezius and rhomboid pedicle, tunneled underneath the paraspinals,

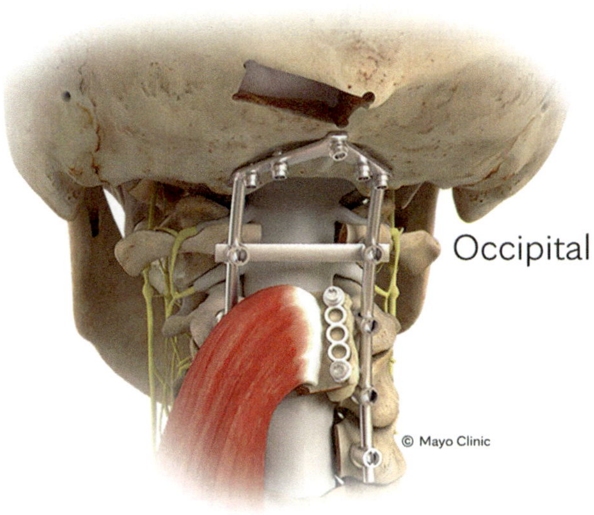

Fig. 10.2 O-VBG extending to cover cervical spinal defect, reproduced with permission from the Mayo Clinic

and the bleeding edge of the bone is articulated directly with the decorticated laminectomy site. Miniplates and screws are used, as with all of the VBG types, to affix the S-VBG accordingly (Fig. 10.3).

The Rib

The R-VBG has been an option in clinical practice for complex spinal reconstruction for many years now, with literature supporting improvement of outcomes for patients, with little increase of operative time and local site morbidity [28, 36, 50–54]. The most common rib of choice due to anatomical location, degree of curvature, and dorsal topography is the eighth rib, which can be utilized for coverage from around C6 to L5 and 16 cm in length. However, using another rib may be considered to better customize the kyphosis/lordosis desired based upon the varying degrees of curvature found in each native rib. A more extensive lateral release may also be required as donor to recipient site and corresponding pedicle lengths are directly correlated. For R-VBG harvest, the surgeon first makes a lateral incision, bluntly dissecting all attachments of the superior border of the rib and carefully dissecting posteriorly away from the pleura. Inferior attachments are left intact with care not to injure the neurovasculature within the costal groove. Distal and proximal bone cuts are made to release the R-VBG. Once hemostasis is achieved, especially in the lateral costal vessels, a lateral release using the subperiosteal technique is made to allow the graft to reach the spinal defect. The longer the muscular pedicle, the greater the extent of lateral release required. The graft is then tunneled underneath the paraspinal muscles to reach the posterolateral gutter, just adjacent to the

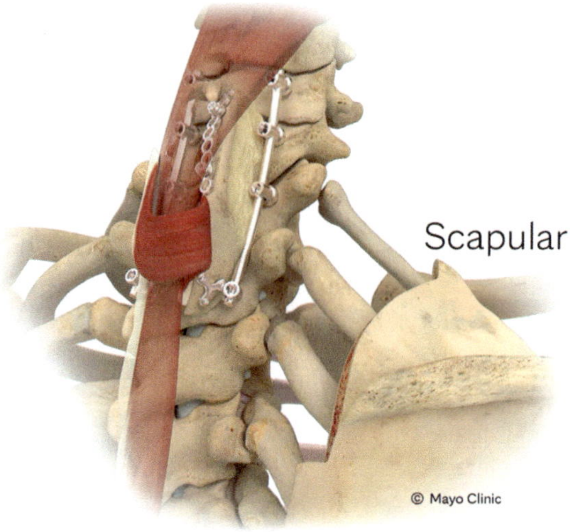

Fig. 10.3 S-VBG utilizing the rhomboid minor and trapezius as the muscular pedicle, reproduced with permission from the Mayo Clinic

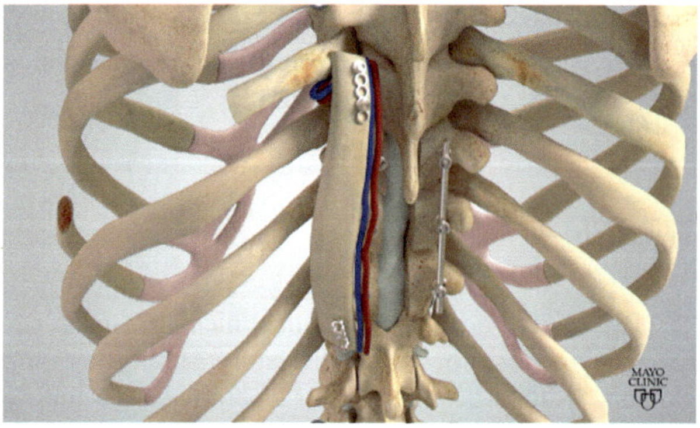

Fig. 10.4 R-VBG taken with the subcostal artery of the eighth rib for augmentation of spinal fusion, reproduced with permission from the Mayo Clinic

laminectomy site at the defect (Fig. 10.4). To lock the graft in place and add compressive force, top-loading rods may be used. It is recommended to perform a bubble test with positive pressure to ensure no pneumothorax has occurred. Medial advancement of the paraspinous muscle then offers more soft tissue coverage prior to layered closure in the usual fashion.

The Clavicle

While posterior approaches have been discussed with prior mentioned VBG types, C-VBGs may be indicated for anterior cervicothoracic spinal defects, particularly those complex cases requiring long-segment ventral reconstruction and with an arc of rotation from C2-T2 and up to 12 cm in length [24, 55]. The procedure requires the standard anterior cervical instrumentation and fusion with the patient in the supine position, head slightly extended. The surgeon's incision is from the level of the hyoid to the sternal notch, along the medial edge of the sternocleidomastoid (SCM). Next, the anterior cervical triangle is exposed by careful dissection of the platysma. Careful dissection and exposure of both sternal and clavicular heads of the SCM, as well as the medial and lateral borders, prepares visualization of the ventral clavicle. Subperiosteal dissection is performed from the lateral edge of the sternoclavicular joint and to the most lateral point of exposure of incision. The superior SCM and inferior pectoralis attachments remain intact throughout. The superior two-thirds of the clavicle is then cut with care to preserve the inferior one-third and the sternoclavicular joint, preventing functional and cosmetic harm. However, if there is a robust graft requirement, removal of the entire clavicular segment may be considered. The superior thyroid and occipital branches supplying the SCM should remain uninjured and adequate for graft viability, despite the disruption of the supraclavicular artery. The C-VBG is rotated on the clavicular head of the SCM until it reaches the level of arthrodesis (Fig. 10.5). The graft is then fixed at the optimal angle to restore native cervical lordosis.

The Spinous Process

After a posterior approach to instrumentation and fusion, further exposure is not required for the harvest of a SP-VBG as it has been described in literature for thoracolumbar reconstruction [56]. Unilaterally, from the spinous process to the facet joints and transverse processes of the fused segment, subperiosteal dissection is performed. Moving to the contralateral side, an effort is made to maintain viable periosteum and paraspinal muscle attachment while the superficial investing fascia is released. The spinous processes of the affected segment are then cut with a drill or osteotome at the base and advanced to the previously decorticated articular and transverse processes. Wire cable or resorbable suture prevents extrusion of the graft, securing the graft within the posterolateral space. Then the standard fascial and multilayered closure can be performed.

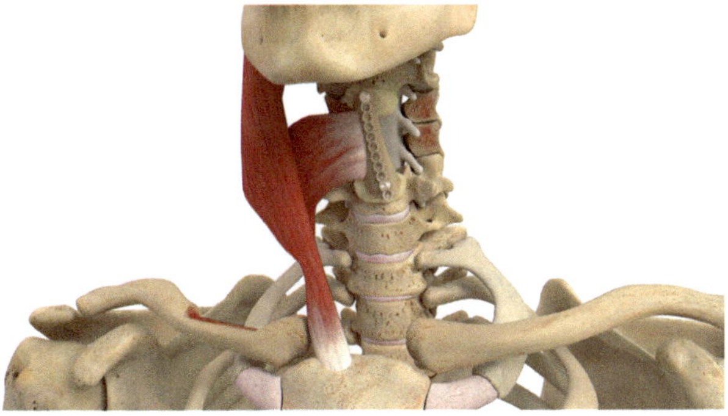

Fig. 10.5 C-VBG with an SCM pedicle, reproduced with permission from the Mayo Clinic

Maximizing Surgical Success

Multidisciplinary and Multifactorial Approach

Teamwork is inherent in spino-plastics. The field itself is built upon collaboration with other spinal surgeons in orthopedics and neurosurgery to provide the best individualized care for each patient. Hence, there is a greater emphasis on the patient selection and preoperative planning aspects of patient care to optimize surgical outcomes. Candidacy for a VBG includes all factors considered for any surgical procedure in addition to the characteristics of the vertebral defect in question: size, length, level, and other native anatomical variables. Once it is determined that a patient is a good candidate for a VBG, then there must be strategic selection of VBG type. One must take into consideration the size, location, and characteristics of the spinal defects, as well as patient factors including comorbidities and prior surgical interventions.

Enhancing Efficiency and Assessing Graft Viability

Intraoperative efficiency necessitates adequate planning, and utilization of VBGs allows for faster operative times as compared to free flaps. Many times, access to the VBG donor site can be gained through extension of existing incision created for instrumentation. This greatly minimizes morbidity. Other strategies for better integration and healing are biologic enhancements and ensuring graft viability prior to placement. If any extra bone is harvested during procurement of the VBG, after it is cut to size, it may then be used as a nonvascularized graft at the area of defect. Graft viability is not always visualized by bleeding at the leading edge. In these circumstances, intraoperative indocyanine green (ICG) fluorescence can be used to assess graft viability. The technique of graft placement and fixation by the plastic surgeon, ensuring direct contact between exposed medullary surfaces, is essential for proper healing and long-term fusion.

Conclusion

Chimeric Flaps: The Road Ahead

Chimeric flaps, which are comprised of separate tissue types or independent territories that may have multiple perforasomes, are employed to address extensive and highly complex defects [57–59]. Multicomponent vascularized grafting restores cosmesis, geometric composition, and quality at the site of deficiency during a single-stage operation [58]. Fixing a bony defect in conjunction with a large soft-tissue lesion is a common problem encountered by craniofacial surgeons, which has created a steady stream of procedural innovation.

VBGs within spino-plastics are a new generation of the musculo-osseous reconstruction traditionally seen in craniofacial literature and practice. Deep circumflex iliac perforator flaps have been used in craniofacial reconstruction for many years, offering superior results to their counterpart grafts that do not have muscle and bone components [60, 61]. Chimeric grafting minimizes residual deficits despite the initially high level of disfiguration described. Like craniofacial defects, spinal defects require special attention to the durability and functionality of surgical outcomes. The field of spino-plastics is a burgeoning field, ripe with investigation of new techniques in graft harvest, placement, and fixation for optimal results.

After numerous VBG cases we have identified that there is an increase in fusion rate, a decrease in time to fusion, and an increased density of ossification in spinal fusion associated with the vascularized bone grafts. This being noted, we anticipate that their use will become more incorporated in primary as well as secondary surgery. The most evident of these would be in scoliosis surgery in which there are significant forces to revert to the scoliosis priority state even after traditional fusion has taken place. We are seeing increasing amounts of vascularized bone grafts used primarily in these cases. It stands to reason that vascularized bone grafts may be standard for all primary spine surgeries that require fusion. Future directions of spino-plastic surgery include understanding the minimal amount of surface area of Sharpey's fibers that are required to support a given distance of vascularized bone. For instance, a one-centimeter insertion of a muscle unit can support a 10-centimeter length of bone; alternatively, can millimeters of Sharpey's fibers support a small bone graft saving the posterior abdominal wall and/or the musculature of the cervical spine?

It is anticipated that there will be an impact on free tissue transfer as well with ideas concerning bone, functional muscle, and bone chimeric free tissue transfer. This concept which becomes apparent with the lowest rib quadratus lumborum iliac crest functional free flap may lead to advances in head and neck or extremity surgeries. This stems from the work with vascularized grafting in the spine.

Spino-plastic surgery has a transformational impact on spine surgery, and we will see expanded uses of VBGs in different areas around the spine; however, we will also see a refinement in an application throughout the body as has previously been noted, such as craniofacial surgery, hand and wrist, and foot and ankle surgery. Further research will stratify the risks of patients who are undergoing spine surgery and identify the best applications for VBGs. There is an ongoing need for innovation in this field to achieve superior surgical outcomes, improving the quality of life for patients undergoing complex spine surgery.

In conclusion, it is necessary to expand the algorithm for complex reconstruction of the spine and surgical planning for these cases. The team-based approach in spino-plastic surgery widened and broadened the capabilities of surgeons to positively affect patient outcomes. This mandates that plastic surgeons innovate and share these techniques across the field of spine surgery in applying VBGs for spinal fusion.

Works Cited

1. Reeg SE. A review of comorbidities and spinal surgery. Clin Orthop Relat Res. 2001;384:101–9.
2. Delancy MM, Perdanasari A, Davis MJ, et al. The advent of spinoplastics: easing the growing global disease burden of spinal injury. Semin Plast Surg. 2021;35:41–9.
3. Reece EM. Spino-plastic reconstruction. Semin Plast Surg. 2021;35:2.
4. Jeger JL, Simoni A, Shvedova M, et al. Spino-plastic surgery: a literature review of vascularized bone grafts and their uses in spine reconstruction. Orthoplastic Surg. 2023;14:15–22.
5. Mobbs RJ, Phan K, Malham G, Seex K, Rao PJ. Lumbar interbody fusion: techniques, indications and comparison of interbody fusion options including PLIF, TLIF, MI-TLIF, OLIF/ATP, LLIF and ALIF. J Spine Surg. 2015;1:2–18.
6. Kumar R, Guinto FC Jr, Madewell JE, Swischuk LE, David R. The vertebral body: radiographic configurations in various congenital and acquired disorders. Radiographics. 1988;8:455–85.
7. Boss S, Srivastava V, Anitescu M. Vertebroplasty and Kyphoplasty. Phys Med Rehabil Clin N Am. 2022;33:425–53.
8. Hoffmann J, Preston G, Whaley J, Khalil JG. Vertebral Augmentation in Spine Surgery. J Am Acad Orthop Surg. 2023;31:477–89.
9. Uppin AA, Hirsch JA, Centenera LV, Pfiefer BA, Pazianos AG, Choi IS. Occurrence of new vertebral body fracture after percutaneous vertebroplasty in patients with osteoporosis. Radiology. 2003;226:119–24.
10. Allain J, Dufour T. Anterior lumbar fusion techniques: ALIF, OLIF, DLIF, LLIF, IXLIF. Orthop Traumatol Surg Res. 2020;106:S149–s57.
11. Matsuyama Y. Surgical treatment for adult spinal deformity: conceptual approach and surgical strategy. Spine Surg Relat Res. 2017;1:56–60.
12. Rajaee SS, Bae HW, Kanim LE, Delamarter RB. Spinal fusion in the United States: analysis of trends from 1998 to 2008. Spine (Phila Pa 1976). 2012;37:67–76.
13. Harris IA, Traeger A, Stanford R, Maher CG, Buchbinder R. Lumbar spine fusion: what is the evidence? Intern Med J. 2018;48:1430–4.
14. Nasser R, Yadla S, Maltenfort MG, et al. Complications in spine surgery. J Neurosurg Spine. 2010;13:144–57.
15. Zuckerman SL, Devin CJ. Pseudarthrosis of the cervical spine. Clin Spine Surg. 2022;35:97–106.
16. How NE, Street JT, Dvorak MF, et al. Pseudarthrosis in adult and pediatric spinal deformity surgery: a systematic review of the literature and meta-analysis of incidence, characteristics, and risk factors. Neurosurg Rev. 2019;42:319–36.
17. Horn SR, Dhillon ES, Poorman GW, et al. Epidemiology and national trends in prevalence and surgical management of metastatic spinal disease. J Clin Neurosci. 2018;53:183–7.
18. Cruz A, Ropper AE, Xu DS, et al. Failure in lumbar spinal fusion and current management modalities. Semin Plast Surg. 2021;35:54–62.
19. Zhang S, Liu Z, Lu C, et al. Oblique lateral interbody fusion combined with different internal fixations for the treatment of degenerative lumbar spine disease: a finite element analysis. BMC Musculoskelet Disord. 2022;23:206.
20. Verla T, Xu DS, Davis MJ, et al. Failure in cervical spinal fusion and current management modalities. Semin Plast Surg. 2021;35:10–3.
21. Sparks DS, Wagels M, Taylor GI. Bone reconstruction: a history of vascularized bone transfer. Microsurgery. 2018;38:7–13.
22. Taylor GI, Miller GD, Ham FJ. The free vascularized bone graft. A clinical extension of microvascular techniques. Plast Reconstr Surg. 1975;55:533–44.
23. Yelizarov VG, Minachenko VK, Gerasimov OR, Pshenisnov KP. Vascularized bone flaps for thoracolumbar spinal fusion. Ann Plast Surg. 1993;31:532–8.
24. Skochdopole AJ, Wagner RD, Davis MJ, et al. Vascularized bone grafts in spinal reconstruction: an overview of nomenclature and indications. Semin Plast Surg. 2021;35:50–3.

25. Gottlieb LJ, Krieger LM. From the reconstructive ladder to the reconstructive elevator. Plast Reconstr Surg. 1994;93:1503–4.
26. Fernandez de Grado G, Keller L, Idoux-Gillet Y, et al. Bone substitutes: a review of their characteristics, clinical use, and perspectives for large bone defects management. J Tissue Eng. 2018;9:2041731418776819.
27. Bohl MA, Reece EM, Farrokhi F, Davis MJ, Abu-Ghname A, Ropper AE. Vascularized bone grafts for spinal fusion-part 3: the occiput. Oper Neurosurg (Hagerstown). 2021;20:502–7.
28. Reece EM, Agrawal N, Wagner KM, et al. Vascularized bone grafts for spinal fusion-part 2: the rib. Oper Neurosurg (Hagerstown). 2021;20:497–501.
29. Reece EM, Davis MJ, Abu-Ghname A, et al. Vascularized bone grafts for spinal fusion-part 4: the scapula. Oper Neurosurg (Hagerstown). 2021;20:508–12.
30. Reece EM, O'Neill RC, Davis MJ, et al. Vascularized scapular bone grafting: indications, techniques, clinical outcomes, and alternatives. Semin Plast Surg. 2021;35:25–30.
31. Shin AY, Dekutoski MB. The role of vascularized bone grafts in spine surgery. Orthop Clin North Am. 2007;38(61–72):vi.
32. Cohen LE, Fullerton N, Mundy LR, et al. Optimizing successful outcomes in complex spine reconstruction using local muscle flaps. Plast Reconstr Surg. 2016;137:295–301.
33. Winters HA, van Engeland AE, Jiya TU, van Royen BJ. The use of free vascularised bone grafts in spinal reconstruction. J Plast Reconstr Aesthet Surg. 2010;63:516–23.
34. Ou Q, Wu P, Zhou Z, Pan D, Tang JY. Complication of osteo reconstruction by utilizing free vascularized fibular bone graft. BMC Surg. 2020;20:216.
35. Soucacos PN, Kokkalis ZT, Piagkou M, Johnson EO. Vascularized bone grafts for the management of skeletal defects in orthopaedic trauma and reconstructive surgery. Injury. 2013;44(Suppl 1):S70–5.
36. Wilden JA, Moran SL, Dekutoski MB, Bishop AT, Shin AY. Results of vascularized rib grafts in complex spinal reconstruction. J Bone Joint Surg Am. 2006;88:832–9.
37. Prablek M, McGinnis J, Winocour SJ, et al. Failures in thoracic spinal fusions and their management. Semin Plast Surg. 2021;35:20–4.
38. Reece EM, Davis MJ, Wagner RD, et al. Vascularized bone grafts for spinal fusion-part 1: the iliac crest. Oper Neurosurg (Hagerstown). 2021;20:493–6.
39. Bohl MA, Hlubek RJ, Turner JD, Reece EM, Kakarla UK, Chang SW. Novel surgical treatment strategies for unstable lumbar osteodiscitis: a 3-patient case series. Oper Neurosurg (Hagerstown). 2018;14:639–46.
40. Bohl MA, Mooney MA, Catapano JS, et al. Pedicled vascularized bone grafts for posterior lumbosacral fusion: a cadaveric feasibility study and case report. Spine Deform. 2018;6:498–506.
41. Sasso RC, LeHuec JC, Shaffrey C. Iliac crest bone graft donor site pain after anterior lumbar interbody fusion: a prospective patient satisfaction outcome assessment. J Spinal Disord Tech. 2005;18(Suppl):S77–81.
42. Winocour SJ, Schultz KP, Davis MJ, et al. Vascularized posterior iliac crest bone grafting: indications, techniques, clinical outcomes, and alternatives. Semin Plast Surg. 2021;35:37–40.
43. Hartman JT, McCarron RF, Robertson WW Jr. A pedicle bone grafting procedure for failed lumbosacral spinal fusion. Clin Orthop Relat Res. 1983:223–7.
44. Sheehan JM, Jane JA. Occipital bone graft for atlantoaxial fusion. Acta Neurochir. 2000;142:661–6; discussion 7.
45. Robertson SC, Menezes AH. Occipital calvarial bone graft in posterior occipitocervical fusion. Spine (Phila Pa 1976). 1998;23:249–54; discussion 54–5.
46. Winocour SJ, Xue EY, Bohl MA, et al. Vascularized occipital bone grafting: indications, techniques, clinical outcomes, and alternatives. Semin Plast Surg. 2021;35:14–9.
47. Bohl MA, Mooney MA, Catapano JS, et al. Pedicled vascularized bone grafts for posterior occipitocervical and cervicothoracic fusion: a cadaveric feasibility study. Oper Neurosurg (Hagerstown). 2018;15:318–24.

48. Thoma A, Archibald S, Payk I, Young JE. The free medial scapular osteofasciocutaneous flap for head and neck reconstruction. Br J Plast Surg. 1991;44:477–82.
49. Kärcher H, Feichtinger M. Transformation of a vascularised iliac crest or scapula bone to a pedicled osteomuscular transplant for reconstruction of distant defects in the head and neck region: a new method of transforming two Island flaps to one longer Island flap. J Craniomaxillofac Surg. 2014;42:2056–63.
50. Lin CH, Wei FC, Levin LS, et al. Free composite serratus anterior and rib flaps for tibial composite bone and soft-tissue defect. Plast Reconstr Surg. 1997;99:1656–65.
51. Bruck JC, Bier J, Kistler D. The serratus anterior osteocutaneous free flap. J Reconstr Microsurg. 1990;6:209–13.
52. Georgescu AV, Ivan O. Serratus anterior-rib free flap in limb bone reconstruction. Microsurgery. 2003;23:217–25.
53. Chen HC, Fallico N, Ciudad P, Trignano E. Latissimus dorsi-rib pedicle flap for mandibular reconstruction as a salvage procedure for failed free fibula flap. J Craniofac Surg. 2014;25:961–3.
54. Ohsumi N, Shimamoto R, Tsukagoshi T. Free composite latissimus dorsi muscle-rib flap not containing the intercostal artery and vein for reconstruction of bone and soft-tissue defects. Plast Reconstr Surg. 1994;94:372–8.
55. Bohl MA, Mooney MA, Catapano JS, et al. Pedicled vascularized clavicular graft for anterior cervical arthrodesis: cadaveric feasibility study, technique description, and case report. Spine (Phila Pa 1976). 2017;42:E1266–e71.
56. Bohl MA, Almefty KK, Preul MC, et al. Vascularized spinous process graft rotated on a paraspinous muscle pedicle for lumbar fusion: technique description and early clinical experience. World Neurosurg. 2018;115:186–92.
57. Hallock GG. The complete nomenclature for combined perforator flaps. Plast Reconstr Surg. 2011;127:1720–9.
58. Huang W-C, Chen H-C, Wei F-C, Cheng M-H, Schnur DP. Chimeric flap in clinical use. Clin Plast Surg. 2003;30:457–67.
59. Raghuram AC, Manfro G, Teixeira Gov, et al. Use of single chimeric free flaps or double free flaps for complex head and neck reconstruction. J Reconstr Microsurg. 2021;37:791–8.
60. Koshima I, Yamamoto H, Hosoda M, Moriguchi T, Orita Y, Nagayama H. Free combined composite flaps using the lateral circumflex femoral system for repair of massive defects of the head and neck regions: an introduction to the chimeric flap principle. Plast Reconstr Surg. 1993;92:411–20.
61. Zhang C, Zeng Y, Zhou L, Tang X. The application of chimeric deep circumflex iliac artery perforator flap for oromandibular reconstruction: a case report. Medicine (Baltimore). 2021;100:e25458.

Index

J. P. Agarwal, D. W. Mathes (eds.), *Bone Flaps in Reconstructive Surgery*, https://doi.org/10.1007/978-3-032-12540-8

GPSR Compliance

The European Union's (EU) General Product Safety Regulation (GPSR) is a set of rules that requires consumer products to be safe and our obligations to ensure this.

If you have any concerns about our products, you can contact us on ProductSafety@springernature.com

In case Publisher is established outside the EU, the EU authorized representative is:

Springer Nature Customer Service Center GmbH
Europaplatz 3
69115 Heidelberg, Germany

Batch number: 10134800

Printed by Printforce, the Netherlands